Manual on
Urogynecology in Limited-Resource Setup

68th All India Congress of Obstetrics & Gynaecology

aicog Delhi 2026

Advocate Innovate Challenge Optimise Globalise

68th All India Congress of Obstetrics & Gynaecology
aicog Delhi 2026
Advocate Innovate Challenge Optimise Globalise

Conference Theme
2026 68th AICOG DELHI All India Congress of Obstetrics & Gynaecology
Inspire, Include, Invent: Improving Women's Health in India

Manual on
Urogynecology in Limited-Resource Setup

Series Editors

Ashok Kumar
MD PhD
Director–Professor
Department of Obstetrics and Gynecology
Atal Bihari Vajpayee Institute of Medical Sciences
and Dr Ram Manohar Lohia Hospital
New Delhi, India

Madhavi M Gupta
MS
Director–Professor
Department of Obstetrics and Gynecology
Maulana Azad Medical College and Lok Nayak Hospital
New Delhi, India

K Aparna Sharma
MBBS MD
Professor
Department of Obstetrics and Gynecology
All India Institute of Medical Sciences
New Delhi, India

Editors

Kavita Barnwal
Amita Jain
Richa Vatsa
Nita Thakre
Rajesh Kumari

JAYPEE

JAYPEE BROTHERS MEDICAL PUBLISHERS
The Health Sciences Publisher
New Delhi | London

Message from Series Editors

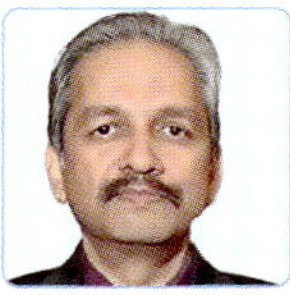

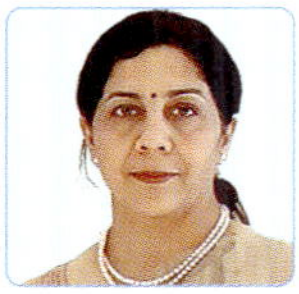

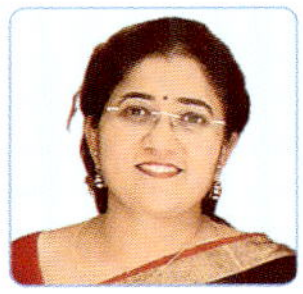

Ashok Kumar
Organizing Chairperson
AICOG-2026
New Delhi

Madhavi M Gupta
Organizing Secretary
AICOG-2026
New Delhi

K Aparna Sharma
Organizing Secretary
AICOG-2026
New Delhi

It is after 18 long years that the 68th AICOG is being held in New Delhi. It is a pleasure to welcome you all.

The Organizing Team have poured their heart and soul into curating an academic program which one will feel a loss if missed. The scientific sessions include both national and international faculty who are stalwarts in their fields. There are 18 workshops with 8 full-day and 5 each in the pre-lunch and post-lunch time.

On this occasion, the workshop faculty, have gone that extra mile to publish the workshop manual for eight workshops. This includes all recent scientific evidence and clinical management guidelines. These manuals will serve as a go-to evidence-based resource in your day-to-day clinical practice. We look forward to receiving your valuable feedback.

We acknowledge the hard work put in by all the editors, co-editors, and the authors, who, in spite of busy schedules and time constraints, have contributed immensely.

We would also like to thank M/s Jaypee Brothers Medical Publishers (P) Ltd, New Delhi, India, for partnering with us.

We sincerely hope that you will enjoy reading these manuals, find this manual useful, and treasure it for future use in your practical work.

We take this opportunity to wish you a memorable time during your stay in New Delhi.

Warm Regards

Jaypee Brothers Medical Publishers (P) Ltd

Headquarters
EMCA House, 23/23-B
Ansari Road, Daryaganj
New Delhi 110 002, India
Landline: +91-11-23272143, +91-11-23272703
+91-11-23282021, +91-11-23245672
e-mail: jaypee@jaypeebrothers.com

Corporate Office
4838/24, Ansari Road, Daryaganj
New Delhi 110 002, India
Phone: +91-11-43574357
Fax: +91-11-43574314
e-mail: jaypee@jaypeebrothers.com

Overseas Office
JP Medical Ltd.
83, Victoria Street, London
SW1H 0HW (UK)
Phone: +44-20 3170 8910
e-mail: info@jpmedpub.com

EU GPSR Authorised Representative
Logos Europe, 9 rue Nicolas Poussin
17000, La Rochelle, France
Phone: +33 (0) 6 67 93 73 78
e-mail: contact@logoseurope.eu

Website: www.jaypeebrothers.com
Website: www.jaypeedigital.com

Inquiries for bulk sales may be solicited at: jaypee@jaypeebrothers.com

Manual on Urogynecology in Limited-Resource Setup

First Edition: **2026**

ISBN: 978-93-7545-652-0

Printed at: Samrat Offset Pvt. Ltd.

Contributors

Amita Jain
MS (Obs & Gyn) Fellowship Urogynaecology,
James Cook University, Australia
Associate Director and Urogynecologist
Institute of Urology and Robotic Surgery
Medanta—The Medicity Hospital
Gurugram, Haryana, India

Jai Bhagwan Sharma MBBS MD
Head
Department of Obstetrics
and Gynecology
Yashoda Medicity
Indirapuram, Ghaziabad, India

Karishma Thariani MBBS MS
Consultant
Department of Obstetrics
and Gynecology
Center for Urogynecology
and Pelvic Health
New Delhi, India

Kavita Barnwal
MBBS (Hon) MS (PMCH) MICOG FICOG
Fertility Specialist
Indira IVF, Samarpan Hospital, Munger
Associate Professor
Department of Obstetrics
and Gynecology
Lord Buddha Koshi Medical College
Saharsa, Bihar, India
Chairperson, Urogynaec Pelvic Floor
Repair Committee

Manasi Deoghare MBBS MD
Department of Obstetrics
and Gynecology
All India Institute of Medical Sciences
New Delhi, India
Fellow, Urogynecology and Pelvic
Reconstructive Surgery

Manidip Pal MBBS MD
Professor and Principal
Department of Obstetrics
and Gynecology
College of Medicine and
JNM Hospital
Kalyani, West Bengal, India

Rajesh Kumari
Additional Professor
Department of Obstetrics
and Gynecology
All India Institute of Medical
Sciences
New Delhi, India

Richa Vatsa
MD DNB MRCOG
Associate professor
Department of Obstetrics
and Gynecology
All India Institute of Medical Sciences
New Delhi, India

Sandhya Jain MD DNB
Department of Obstetrics
and Gynecology
All India Institute of Medical
Sciences
New Delhi, India
Director and Professor
University College of Medical Sciences
and GTB Hospital
New Delhi, India

Soma Bandyopadhyay
MBBS MD
Professor and Head
Katihar Medical College
Al-Karim University
Katihar, Bihar, India

Preface

Female urogynecology care is essential for improving quality-of-life by addressing conditions such as incontinence, prolapse, genitourinary syndrome of menopause, fistulas, etc. Quietly, often invisibly, urogynecological disorders shape the daily lives of countless women. Long after childbirth or surgery, and sometimes without any obvious trigger, symptoms such as incontinence, prolapse, fistula, etc., erode comfort, confidence, and dignity. These conditions may not be life-threatening, yet they profoundly affect quality-of-life—and when neglected, their burden deepens over time. Timely evaluation and appropriate management restore dignity, physical comfort, and social well-being, reduce long-term complications, and empower women to seek care without stigma or disability.

This workshop manual has been developed as a practical and academic guide for clinicians committed to restoring function, dignity, and well-being in women with urogynecological disorders, particularly within limited-resource settings. It acknowledges a crucial reality: effective urogynecological care does not always depend on advanced technology, but on sound clinical judgment, anatomical understanding, and thoughtful, timely intervention.

The focus of this manual is grounded in real-world practice. It addresses common yet challenging conditions through rational evaluation, context-appropriate decision-making, and adaptable surgical techniques. Emphasis is placed on prevention of complications, safe execution of procedures, and the ability to manage adverse outcomes with confidence.

What distinguishes this initiative is its commitment to transforming knowledge into capability. Each section is designed to move beyond theory, fostering practical insight, surgical preparedness, and reflective practice. The workshop format encourages hands-on learning, shared experience, and collaborative problem-solving, reinforcing that excellence in urogynecology is built through collective wisdom and continual refinement of skills.

As caregivers to women across all stages of life, our responsibility extends beyond treatment to restoration—of function, comfort, and self-worth. It is our hope that this manual will sharpen clinical acumen, inspire thoughtful action, and strengthen the resolve to deliver compassionate, effective urogynecological care.

Because when we address urogynecological health with skill and sensitivity, we do more than treat a condition—we restore dignity.

Editors: **Kavita Barnwal, Amita Jain, Richa Vatsa, Nita Thakre, Rajesh Kumari**

Contents

1 CHAPTER

Urinary Incontinence: Evaluation and Initial Workup

Rajesh Kumari, Manasi Deoghare

INTRODUCTION

Urinary incontinence (UI) defined by International Continence Society as complaint of involuntary loss of urine. It affects physical health, quality of life, sexual function, and causes overall morbidity. Prevalence in nonpregnant women aged >20 years varies between 10 and 60%, exceeding 50–70% in women aged >60 years. Primary categories are stress UI (SUI), urgency (UUI), mixed UI (MUI), and overflow UI. Stress incontinence is defined as incontinence with activities causing increased intraabdominal pressure such as coughing, sneezing, laughing, and exercising and is the most common type of incontinence with peak incidence in younger and middle age groups. Urgency urinary incontinence is involuntary leakage of urine associated with sudden, compelling desire to void that is difficult to defer. It is more prevalent in older women. Mixed incontinence is when women have symptoms of both stress and urgency. Overflow incontinence occurs in presence of excessively full bladder and results in continuous urinary leakage.

EVALUATION OF URINARY INCONTINENCE

- *History*: A thorough history is essential for diagnosing urinary incontinence. It should include following points:
    - Characterization of incontinence (e.g., stress, urgency, mixed, continuous, and without sensory awareness)
    - Chronicity of symptoms
    - Frequency, bother, and severity of incontinence episodes
    - Patient's expectations of treatment (e.g., patient centered goals)
    - Pad or protection use
    - Other lower urinary tract symptoms (e.g., urgency, frequency, nocturia, dysuria, hematuria, slow flow, hesitancy, and incomplete emptying)
    - Volume and type of fluid intake (e.g., coffee, tea, and alcohol)
    - Other pelvic symptoms (e.g., pelvic pain, pressure, bulging, and dyspareunia)
    - Gastrointestinal symptoms (e.g., constipation, diarrhea, and splinting to defecate)

- Obstetric history (e.g., gravity, parity, method of delivery, episiotomy, and baby weight)
- Previous incontinence treatments or surgery (e.g., behavioral therapy, Kegel exercises/pelvic floor muscle training, pharmacotherapy, and surgery)
- Previous pelvic surgeries
- Present and past medical history (e.g., hypertension, diabetes, and history of pelvic radiation)
- Current and past medications—fluid, alcohol, and caffeine intake
- Menopausal status

▪ Symptom questionnaires should be used determine the presence of UI and delve into the specifics of degree, bother, and subtype and the effect on quality of life. The commonly used questionnaires are ICIQ-UI Short Form, ICIQ-FLUTS, ICIQ-MLUTS, IIQ and IIQ-7, I-QOL, KHQ, PFDI-20, etc.

▪ *Bladder diary:* Three day bladder diary provides vital information about the volume and type of fluid intake, the number of voids, bladder capacity as assessed for the volume of voids, degree of urgency associated with voids, number of incontinence episodes and the reason for incontinence (urge, cough, laugh, exercise, etc.)

▪ Physical examination should include the following components:
- Focused abdominal examination
- Supine and/or standing stress test with comfortably full bladder, if positive, empty bladder leak test can be done if intrinsic sphincter deficiency is suspected
- Q tip test is a test to see urethral hypermobility in cases of SUI done by placing a cotton swab through the urethral meatus to bladder neck and measuring the displacement. If >30°, suggestive of urethral hypermobility. Not recommended to diagnose SUI and does not correlate with urethral function tests in urodynamics.
- *Bonney test:* On lifting the paraurethral tissues with middle and index finger, if no leaks with cough, considered as a positive Bonney test and suggestive of urethral hypermobility and likely success of colposuspension procedures. The relevance of this test has diminished because there is lack of standardization and often works by artificial compression and obstruction of the urethra giving false positive report.
- Assessment of pelvic prolapse (if any)
- Assessment of vaginal atrophy/estrogenization status
- Look for sequalae of urinary incontinence like skin rash, excoriation, or ulceration
- Assessment of pelvic floor muscles and ability to perform Kegel exercise

    - Focused neurologic examination
    - Observation of patient's gait to help identify mobility impairments
- Diagnostic evaluations that should be performed include following:
    - *Urinalysis*: Consideration of the correlation between incomplete bladder voiding and urinary tract infections (UTIs) should be taken into account. A urinalysis (dipstick or microscopy) should be performed in all patients with urinary incontinence. Urine culture should be performed if urinalysis suggestive of UTI (e.g., nitrites, leukocyte esterase or bacteriuria, pyuria or hematuria).
    - *Post-void residual (PVR)*: Post-void residual volume is the amount of urine that remains in the bladder after voiding. It indicates poor voiding efficiency, which may result from a number of contributing factors. It is important because it may worsen symptoms and, more rarely, may be associated with UTI, upper urinary tract (UUT) dilatation, and renal insufficiency.

      A persistently elevated PVR does not signify the etiology of impaired voiding, but rather necessitates further assessment. An increased PVR could suggest bladder hypocontractility, predisposing a patient to post-treatment retention in cases of SUI. So an elevated PVR may influence patient counselling with regard to surgical interventions and outcome expectations.

      Post-void residual can be measured using ultrasound (preferred) and catheterization. It should be measured within 5–10 minutes of voiding to prevent erroneous reporting of high PVR. Though definite cutoffs are not available for elevated PVR, value <50 mL is considered normal and >150 mL is suggestive of elevated PVR. The test should be repeated when a single abnormally high value is obtained.

      An elevated postvoid residual urine volume in the absence of pelvic organ prolapse is uncommon and should trigger an evaluation of the bladder-emptying mechanism, usually with a pressure-flow urodynamic study.
    - *USG KUB*: Not routinely done. Done in cases of recurrent UTI, hematuria in absence of infection on urinalysis, or neurogenic lower urinary tract dysfunction.
    - *Uroflowmetry and urodynamics study (UDS)*: Uroflowmetry is a noninvasive measurement of flow rate of external urine stream as volume per unit time in milliliters per second. It is indicated in women with urinary incontinence having voiding dysfunction.

      Urodynamics study is an invasive test having two parts: Filling cystometry and pressure flow studies of voiding. It is not necessary in patients with pure SUI and no other urinary symptoms or to predict outcomes after surgery. But UDS should be performed in patients with SUI before surgery in cases of:

- History of prior anti-incontinence surgery
- History of prior pelvic organ prolapse surgery
- Mismatch between subjective and objective measures
- Significant voiding dysfunction
- Significant urgency, UUI, and overactive bladder (OAB)
- Elevated PVR per clinician judgment
- Unconfirmed SUI
- Neurogenic lower urinary tract dysfunction

In cases of overactive bladder and urge urinary incontinence, UDS is indicated in:

- Diagnostic uncertainty
- Mixed incontinence or insensate incontinence
- Obstructive voiding symptoms (e.g., LUTS after sling surgery)
- Neurologic diagnosis/possible neurogenic lower urinary tract dysfunction
- Elevated PVR (as a part of initial evaluation or found after starting OAB therapy)
- Poor response to therapy

- *Cystoscopy*: Not routinely done. Indications are as follows:
  - Cases of UUI and SUI if there is prior sling surgery for SUI.
  - Women with microhematuria in absence of infection
  - Structural urinary tract abnormalities suspected

CONCLUSION

Urinary incontinence is a clinical diagnosis and thorough history and examination are essential before any treatment. Bladder diary and various questionnaires can be used for objectifying and better understanding of patients' symptoms and affection of quality of life. Urinalysis and PVR measurement should be done in all patients and upper tract imaging, urodynamics study and cystoscopy should be done only when indicated.

KEY POINTS

A good detailed history and examination are mandatory in all patients of urinary incontinence to identify the type of incontinence and for further management. Associated findings of voiding dysfunction, bowel complaints, chronic pelvic pain, and prolapse should be noted in all patients. Bladder diary and various questionnaires play a vital role in workup of the patient and urinalysis and PVR should be done in all cases. Upper tract imaging (USG KUB), uroflowmetry, urodynamics study and cystoscopy should be done routinely.

SUGGESTED READING

1. ACOG Practice Bulletin No. 155: Urinary Incontinence in Women. Obstet Gynecol. 2015;126(5):e66-81.

2. Cameron AP, Chung DE, Dielubanza EJ, Enemchukwu E, Ginsberg DA, Helfand BT, et al. The AUA/SUFU Guideline on the Diagnosis and Treatment of Idiopathic Overactive Bladder. J Urol. 2024;212(1):11-20.
3. D'Ancona C, Haylen B, Oelke M, Abranches-Monteiro L, Arnold E, Goldman H, et al. The International Continence Society (ICS) report on the terminology for adult male lower urinary tract and pelvic floor symptoms and dysfunction. Neurourol Urodyn. 2019;38(2):433-77.
4. Kobashi KC, Vasavada S, Bloschichak A, Hermanson L, Kaczmarek J, Kim SK, et al. Updates to Surgical Treatment of Female Stress Urinary Incontinence (SUI): AUA/SUFU Guideline (2023). J Urol. 2023;209(6):1091-8.
5. Lee UJ, Feinstein L, Ward JB, Kirkali Z, Martinez-Miller EE, Matlaga BR, et al. Prevalence of Urinary Incontinence among a Nationally Representative Sample of Women, 2005-2016: Findings from the Urologic Diseases in America Project. J Urol. 2021;205(6):1718-24.
6. Nambiar AK, Bosch R, Cruz F, Lemack GE, Thiruchelvam N, Tubaro A, et al. EAU Guidelines on Assessment and Nonsurgical Management of Urinary Incontinence. Eur Urol. 2018;73(4):596-609.
7. Robledo D, Zuluaga L, Bravo-Balado A, Domínguez C, Trujillo CG, Caicedo JI, et al. Present value of the Urethral mobility test as a tool to assess Stress urinary incontinence due to Intrinsic sphincteric deficiency. Sci Rep. 2020;10(1):20993.

CHAPTER 2

Management of Uterine Prolapse: Knowledge versus Action

Kavita Barnwal

INTRODUCTION

- Pelvic organ prolapse (POP) is a heterogenous condition in which weakness of pelvic floor musculature and connective tissue occurs resulting in descent or bulging of pelvic organs into the vaginal canal **(Fig. 1)**. POP is considered as one of the most common cause of reproductive health morbidity which influences the women's quality of life. This is found more commonly among elderly women.
- The exact prevalence is not available as majority of them do not seek medical help because of social stigma.
- Though prolapse is not life-threatening condition, but it affects women physically, psychologically, sexually and leads to social and occupational limitations. It also increases risk of UTI and reproductive infection.
- UNFPA 2011 describes uterine prolapse as debilitating condition in which supportive pelvic muscles, ligaments and tissue give away and uterus drops into vagina.

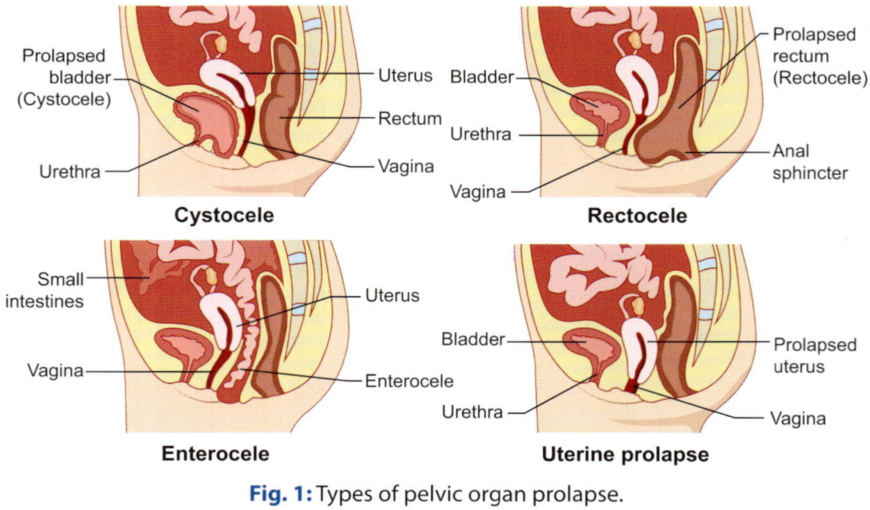

Fig. 1: Types of pelvic organ prolapse.

Anterior wall **Aa**	Anterior wall **Ba**	Cervix or cuff **C**
Genital hiatus **GH**	Perineal body **PB**	Total vaginal length **TVL**
Posterior wall **Ap**	Posterior wall **Bp**	Posterior fornix **D**

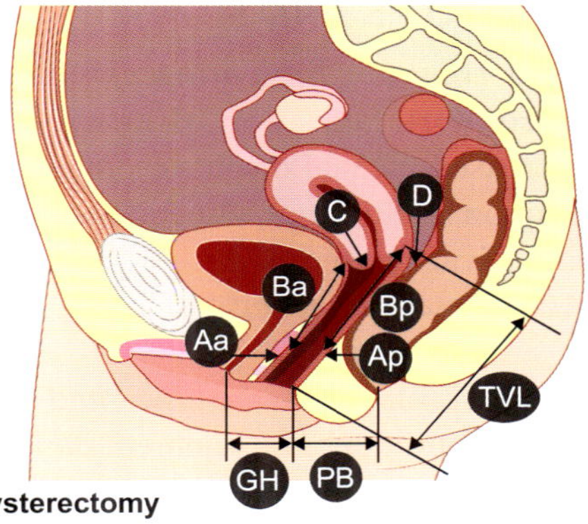

Posthysterectomy

Fig. 2: Pelvic organ prolapse quantification (POP-Q).

CLASSIFICATION OF PROLAPSE

- *Anterior vaginal wall prolapse*: Cystocele and urethrocele
- *Apical prolapse*: Uterine or vault prolapse
- *Post vaginal wall prolapse*: Rectocele and enterocele

Most precise classification is POP-Q quantification **(Fig. 2)**.

Stage 0: No prolapse.

Stage I: The most distal part of the prolapse is >1 cm above the hymen.

Stage II: The most distal part of the prolapse is between 1 cm above and 1 cm below the hymen.

Stage III: The most distal part of the prolapse is >1 cm below the hymen but not past the hymen by 2 cm.

Stage IV: Complete eversion (prolapse) of the vagina.

ETIOLOGY

There are several factors which contribute to weakening of pelvic floor muscles and lead to prolapse:

- Mismanagement or improper care during delivery
- Loss of muscle tone as the result of aging
- Injury during childbirth, especially among multipara
- Delivery of macrosomic fetus
- Obesity
- Chronic cough
- Chronic constipation

All of these factors put added tension on the pelvic muscles, and may contribute to the development of uterine prolapse.

SYMPTOMS AND SIGNS

- *Most common presenting complaint:* Vaginal bulge, pressure, and discomfort, sensation of heaviness in the pelvis, vaginal bleeding, increased vaginal discharge, dyspareunia, low backache, feeling like a tampon is falling out, difficult bowel movements, sexual dysfunction, and lack of vaginal sensation.
- *Associated symptoms:* Relating to voiding, defecation, and sexual dysfunction.
- Uterine prolapse can be prevented and treated depending on the severity of the condition. Management depends on the woman's general health, age, and desire to have children. There are different ways to treat uterine prolapse. First and second degree prolapse can be treated with ring pessaries, which stretches the vaginal walls, often in combination with pelvic floor exercises. Third degree prolapse requires surgical interference.

KNOWLEDGE VERSUS ACTION IN MANAGEMENT OF PROLAPSE

Refers to a common theme in medical and public health literature that there is significant gap between women's knowledge of pelvic organ prolapse and their actual adoption of preventive or management practices.

Studies find that many women have poor knowledge of risk factors, preventive measures, and available treatment options. Some of them do not translate this knowledge into practice due to economic, social, and psychological barriers. Asymptomatic prolapse is common. Many women have some degree of POP that is not bothersome and does not require invasive treatment. Education and reassurance are appropriate.

Conservative options are first-line treatment. Lifestyle modifications and PFMT can alleviate symptoms and prevent progression in mild to moderate cases.

Vaginal pessaries are durable and effective nonsurgical option with satisfactory results in selected cases of POP.

For symptomatic cases, surgery is advised if conservative measures fail. Decision must be based on discussion of risks, benefits, and patient preferences for preservation of uterus.

During surgical management, ensuring proper apical support is cornerstone of success and helps in preventing recurrence.

THE KNOWLEDGE ACTION GAP

The challenge lies in consistently applying this knowledge.

- *Poor awareness:* Majority of women have little knowledge about the disease, risk factors, symptoms, and complications of uterine prolapse.
- *Inadequate knowledge:* In a study group of women, 93% had no idea about regular Kegel exercises, taking a balanced diet, having regular

bowel habits, avoiding lifting heavy objects, and seeking medical advice for prolonged coughing. Some women think that lifting heavy objects are risk but cannot avoid due to lifestyle or work demands.

- *Mismatch of symptoms and treatment:* Many women think that uterine prolapse is common phenomenon after menopause. There can be disconnect between anatomical severity of prolapse and actual symptoms a woman experiences.
- *Low healthcare seeking behavior:* Some women who develop symptoms, care seeking behavior is often low due to embarrassment, social stigma, lack of time, financial constraints, or a preference for traditional treatment.

MANAGEMENT AND ACTIONABLE STEPS

Effective knowledge for management centers on a comprehensive understanding of the condition and available evidence based treatment. It relies on both preventive and therapeutic aspects.

Preventive Measures (Knowledge to Action)

A key action gap is the insufficient management of underlying modifiable risk factors which are essential for long-term management and prevention.

- *Conservative management*:
    - Lifestyle modification
    - Weight reduction
    - Following a high fiber diet and adequate fluid intake to prevent constipation and straining
    - Avoid heavy lifting
    - Treatment of chronic constipation
    - Consult physician for chronic cough
    - Quit smoking
- *Physical therapy*: Pelvic floor muscle training (PFMT): Kegel exercises during and after pregnancy to strengthen levator ani and supportive muscles.

If done under guidance of physiotherapist, can improve symptoms and, in some cases, the objective severity of the prolapse.

Ensure Skilled Birth Attendance during Labor

Regular antenatal and postnatal checkups with Kegel exercise and proper postnatal rest.

- *Pessaries*: These are highly effective, durable silicone devices inserted into the vagina to provide mechanical support to the pelvic organs. They are good option for women who prefer to avoid surgery or are not fit for surgery with high success rates.
- *Surgery*: Surgical intervention is an option when conservative methods fail or symptoms significantly affect quality of life. The choice of surgery is

highly individualized, considering the patient's age, desire for future pregnancy/sexual function, and overall health. Uterine sparing surgery like sacrohysteropexy and hysterectomy with pelvic floor repair are two options.

- *Action gap*: Converting knowledge into effective practice

The difference between simply knowing the facts and effective management lies in targeted actions by both patients and healthcare providers. While clinicians understand the options, effectively communicating in a way that empowers patient self-management and informed decision making remains a challenge.

Patient Actions

- *Seek care early*: Women should not consider POP a normal part of aging. They should not feel shame or embarrassed. Early consultation allows for more conservative and less invasive management options.
- *Adhere to lifestyle changes*: Actively managing weight, treating constipation with high-fiber diets and fluids, avoiding heavy lifting, and quitting smoking are crucial actions to reduce intra-abdominal pressure.
- *Consistency with PFMT and pessary care*: Regular adherence to prescribed pelvic floor exercises and routine cleaning/follow-up for pessaries are vital for long-term success and to prevent complications.
- Healthcare provider actions
- *Promote education and awareness*: Clinicians need to ensure women are fully informed about conservative treatment options as first-line measures. Prolapse-related knowledge is often low among women seeking care.
- *Implement shared decision-making (SDM)*: Management requires an individualized, patient-centric approach that considers the woman's goals and expectations. Health personnel have a role to help women to express their needs without fear and explain the importance for appropriate preventive measures and treatment in early stage.

  Ultimately, bridging the gap between clinical knowledge of management options active, informed patient engagement, and timely intervention is essential for improving quality of life for women with prolapse.
- *Factors influencing knowledge/practice*: Educational status, family income, and access to antenatal/postnatal care visits are often significantly associated with better knowledge and practices.
- *Physician knowledge and attitudes*: Studies also show that while most doctors are aware of the role of physiotherapy and other treatments, postgraduate doctors tend to advise surgical options more frequently than graduates.

Management Actions versus Information

Management of uterine prolapse involves both conservative (nonsurgical) and surgical options, tailored to the individual patient's symptoms and lifestyle. Knowledge empowers patients to discuss these options and participate actively in their care.

Message: Women have poor knowledge regarding uterine prolapse. Therefore, health education programs regarding uterine prolapse should target women at all places, age groups, and educational levels at rural and urban areas. In addition, health workers should be provided with training to be able to detect cases of uterine prolapse in early stages.

KEY POINTS

Pelvic organ prolapse is a common yet underreported condition resulting from weakening of pelvic floor muscles and connective tissue, leading to descent of pelvic organs into the vaginal canal. Although not life-threatening, POP significantly impacts women's physical comfort, psychological well-being, sexual health, social functioning, and increases the risk of urinary and reproductive tract infections. Its prevalence is higher among elderly and multiparous women, but social stigma and low health-seeking behavior contribute to underdiagnosis. POP is classified anatomically into anterior, apical, and posterior compartment defects, with POP-Q being the most precise staging system. Risk factors include childbirth-related trauma, aging, obesity, chronic cough, constipation, and heavy lifting. Management requires bridging the gap between knowledge and action through patient education, early recognition, and individualized care. Conservative measures such as lifestyle modification, pelvic floor muscle training, and pessaries are first-line options, while surgery is reserved for symptomatic or advanced cases. Effective management relies on shared decision-making, preventive strategies, and timely intervention to improve quality of life.

SUGGESTED READING

1. Aki O, Ibrahim H, Mamdouh H. Perceived Reproductive Morbidity and Treatment Seeking Behavior among ever Married Women in Siwa Oasis, Egypt. J Am Sci. 2011;7(6):749.
2. Detollenaere RJ, den Boon J, Stekelenburg J, Alhafidh AH, Hakvoort RA, Vierhout ME, et al. Treatment of uterine prolapse stage 2 or higher: a randomized multicenter trial comparing sacrospinous fixation with vaginal hysterectomy (SAVE U trial). BMC Womens Health. 2011;11:4.
3. Roos AM, Thakar R, Sultan AH, Burger CW, Paulus AT. Pelvic floor dysfunction: women's sexual concerns unraveled. J Sex Med. 2014;11(3):743-52.
4. Segesten K. Nepales Women Suffering from Uterine Prolapse. A participant Observational Study in A maternity Hospital in Nepal. Sweden: Institute of Medicine, University of Gothenburg; 2012.
5. Shrestha B. Challenges in prevention and timely care of uterine prolapse in Nepal. Sweden: Institute of Medicine, University of Gothenburg; 2015.
6. Tamrakar A. Prevalence of Uterine Prolapse and its Associated Factors in Kaski District of Nepal. JHAS. 2012;2(1):38-41.
7. Thapa B, Rana G, Gurung S. Contributing factors of utero-vaginal prolapse among women attended in Bharatpur Hospital. J Chitwan Med Coll. 2014;4(9):38-42.
8. United Nations Population Fund. Maternal Morbidity Statistics by Region and by Country. New York: United Nations Population Fund; 2011.

3 CHAPTER

Surgical Management of Nulliparous Prolapse

Kavita Barnwal

INTRODUCTION

Pelvic organ prolapse (POP) affects millions of women around the world, with age-standardized prevalence rates of 2,769 per 100,000 women in 2021. Although it greatly affects quality of life (QoL), only 18–50% of women experiencing this issue seek medical attention, largely due to a lack of knowledge, misunderstandings about the condition, and obstacles to accessing health care.

CONSIDERATIONS FOR YOUNG WOMEN

- *Future fertility:* Procedures like sacrospinous hysteropexy allow for future pregnancies.
- *Sexual function:* Reconstructive surgeries aim to maintain or restore normal anatomy, crucial for sexually active women.
- *Mesh use*: While effective, mesh has risks (pain, mesh migration, and need for removal); newer approaches favor abdominal mesh placement (less complication risk) or nonmesh techniques where possible, with careful patient counselling.
- *Minimally invasive (laparoscopic/robotic):* Preferred for faster recovery and less pain.

SURGICAL GOALS

- *Reconstruction*: Restoring pelvic anatomy for long-term support.
- *Durability*: Achieving a lasting repair.
- *Preservation*: Maintaining uterus (if desired) and sexual function.

KEY SURGICAL APPROACHES FOR YOUNG WOMEN

Anterior compartment prolapse (cystocele).

SURGICAL TREATMENT OPTION

- Native tissue suture plication
- Vaginal repair augmented with permanent synthetic mesh (polypropylene)
- Biological graft (treated pig skin or bovine small intestine)

2016 Cochrane review on the surgical management of anterior compartment prolapsed reported the following:

- Synthetic mesh was associated with improved anatomical and subjective outcomes when compared to AC, importantly these outcomes did not translate into improved functional outcomes using validated questionnaires or a lower reoperation rate for prolapse.
- Synthetic mesh was also associated with longer operating time, greater blood loss and higher rate of cystotomy, de-novo SUI, and prolapse of the apical or posterior vaginal compartment.

POSTERIOR COMPARTMENT REPAIR (RECTOCELE)

- Transvaginal options for the repair of posterior vaginal wall defects include midline fascial suture plication [posterior colporrhaphy (PC)], or augmentation of the repair with biological graft or synthetic mesh.
- DeLorme's procedure is a transanal procedure for rectal prolapse but has been evaluated for management of rectocele.
- Ventral rectopexy is an abdominal intervention recommended for rectal prolapse that some have suggested may also be suitable for rectocele.

Findings of the 2017 ICI review include the following:

- PC has superior anatomical success to transanal repair with similar functional outcomes
- No evidence demonstrates benefit for synthetic or biological graft at vaginal repair
- No data demonstrate ventral rectopexy ± vaginal graft is effective for rectocele

Apical suspension procedures can broadly be separated into those performed transvaginally and those performed abdominally.

- Abdominal procedures, including SC or uterosacral ligament suspension, can be performed via laparotomy or using conventional laparoscopic or robotically assisted-laparoscopic techniques.
- Transvaginal apical suspension procedures include native tissue repair (uterosacral and sacrospinous colpopexy) and mesh/graft repairs.
- Sacrocolpopexy (SC) is the preferred apical suspending procedure over the transvaginal native tissue and mesh repairs for vaginal vault prolapse.
- SC has significant anatomical and functional advantages when compared with a broad group of vaginal surgeries (±mesh).
- Vaginal uterosacral and sacrospinous colpopexy are effective vaginal interventions.

ROBOTIC SURGERY

Often robotic-assisted sacrocervicopexy/colpopexy is considered a gold standard for severe prolapse due to precision, durability, and faster recovery.

WHEN TO CHOOSE WHAT

- *Severe prolapse*: Robotic/laparoscopic sacrocolpopexy is often favored.
- *Uterine preservation needed*: Sacrohysteropexy or vaginal hysteropexy options are key.
- *Less invasive/fertility focus*: Vaginal sacrospinous procedures are excellent.

Always discuss these options with a urogynecologist to tailor the best approach, considering the type/severity of prolapse, age, and future goals.

RECONSTRUCTIVE PATHWAY

Majority of women undergoing surgery for POP will undergo reconstructive surgery that aims to address defects:

- Anterior compartment (bladder and urethra)
- Posterior compartment (perineum rectocele or enterocele)
- There is growing recognition that adequate support for the vaginal apex is an essential component of a durable surgical repair for women with advanced prolapse.
- Eiber et al. demonstrated that the reoperation rates for recurrent prolapse 10 years after index surgery were halved in women who underwent apical support procedures at the time of repairs as compared to those with vaginal repair without apical support
- Uterine preservation

RELATIVE CONTRAINDICATIONS

Abnormalities of the uterus (fibroids, adenomyosis, endometrial pathology, abnormal cervical cytology, uterine or postmenopausal bleeding) or factors that increase the risk of gynecological cancer (familial cancer *BRCA1* and *BRCA2* gene, Lynch syndrome, tamoxifen therapy, obesity, and those not compliant with gynecological surveillance).

Many women prefer to keep their uterus for sense of identity, future pregnancy, and concerns about the potential adverse effects of hysterectomy.

Studies indicate that uterine-preserving surgeries (hysteropexy) have success and recurrence rates that are comparable to, and sometimes better than, those involving hysterectomy.

Surgical benefits: Uterus-sparing procedures are associated with benefits such as shorter operating times, less blood loss, and reduced hospital stays.

KEY POINTS

Surgical management of pelvic organ prolapse in nulliparous and young women demands a highly individualized, evidence-based approach that prioritizes long-term anatomical durability while preserving fertility, sexual function, and body integrity. Despite its significant impact on quality of life, prolapse in this population remains under-recognized and undertreated due to poor awareness and delayed healthcare seeking. The primary goal of surgery is anatomical reconstruction with robust apical support, as failure to address the apex is associated with high recurrence rates. Uterus-preserving procedures such as sacrohysteropexy, sacrospinous hysteropexy, and uterosacral ligament suspension have emerged as effective options with outcomes comparable to hysterectomy-based repairs and added benefits of reduced morbidity. Minimally invasive and robotic approaches offer superior visualization, precision, faster recovery, and excellent functional outcomes. The use of mesh requires careful patient selection and counselling, balancing anatomical success against potential complications. Shared decision-making, patient preferences, and future reproductive goals remain central to achieving optimal outcomes in young women with prolapse.

SUGGESTED READING

1. Abrams P, Cardozo L, Wagg A, Wein A (Eds). Incontinence. 6th edition. Tokyo: International Continence Society; 2017.
2. Barber MD, Maher C. Apical prolapse. Int Urogynecol J. 2013;24(11):1815-33.
3. Culligan PJ, Salamon C. A randomized controlled trial comparing robotic-assisted sacrocolpopexy and laparoscopic sacrocolpopexy. Int Urogynecol J. 2012;23(7):915-20.
4. Dietz HP, Maher C. Pelvic organ prolapse and sexual function. Int Urogynecol J. 2013;24(11):1853-7.
5. Diwadkar GB, Barber MD, Feiner B, et al. Complication and reoperation rates after apical vaginal prolapse surgical repair: a systematic review. Obstet Gynecol. 2009;113(2 Pt 1):367-73.
6. Eilber KS, Alperin M, Khan A, et al. Outcomes of vaginal prolapse surgery among women with and without apical support. Am J Obstet Gynecol. 2013;208(6):e1-e7.
7. Haylen BT, de Ridder D, Freeman RM, et al. An International Urogynecological Association (IUGA)/International Continence Society (ICS) joint report on the terminology for female pelvic organ prolapse. Neurourol Urodyn. 2010;29(1):4-20.
8. Maher C, Feiner B, Baessler K, Schmid C. Surgical management of pelvic organ prolapse in women. Cochrane Database Syst Rev. 2013;(4):CD004014.
9. Nygaard I, Brubaker L, Zyczynski HM, et al. Long-term outcomes following abdominal sacrocolpopexy for pelvic organ prolapse. JAMA. 2013;309(19):2016-24.
10. U.S. Food and Drug Administration. Urogynecologic surgical mesh: update on the safety and effectiveness of transvaginal placement for pelvic organ prolapse. Silver Spring (MD): FDA; 2011.

4 CHAPTER

High Uterosacral Ligament Suspension

Manidip Pal, Soma Bandyopadhyay

INTRODUCTION

Uterosacral ligament is one of the very strong ligament of women body. It runs from posterior aspect of lower part of the uterus to anterior aspect of sacrum. It is also known as sacrouterine ligament. One of the very interesting property of uterosacral ligament is that it does not get attenuated with aging process. This property has made it a very good choice for surgical creation of suspension for DeLancey's level 1 support.

Uterosacral ligament is about 12–14 cm in length and divided in three parts—cervical, intermediate, and sacral **(Table 1)**.

Pelvic part of ureter lies laterally along the uterosacral ligament **(Table 2)**.

The uterosacral ligament can hold a weight approximately 17 kg at intermediate and cervical area and about 5 kg at sacral area.

Looking at the anatomical relationship it is understandable that intermediate portion of the uterosacral ligament would be the best area to use for suspension. Hence this is known as high uterosacral ligament suspension (HULS).

Depending on the approach it is of two types:

1. Intraperitoneal HULS
2. Extraperitoneal HULS

TABLE 1: Dimensions of uterosacral ligament.

Parts	*Length (cm)*	*Breadth (cm)*
Cervical	2–3	2 ± 0.5
Intermediate	5	2.7 ± 1
Sacral	5–6	5.2 ± 0.9

TABLE 2: Distance between pelvic part of ureter and uterosacral ligament.

Part of uterosacral ligament	*Distance from ureter (cm)*
Cervical	0.9 ± 0.4
Intermediate	2.3 ± 0.9
Sacral	4.1 ± 0.6

INTRAPERITONEAL HULS

This operation can be traced back to Miller, Heaney, TeLinde, and many others. But it is popularized by Professor Bob Louis Shull of USA.

Procedure (in case of vault prolapse repair):

- Allis forceps are used to hold the vault's apex while an inverted "T" incision is made there.
- The vaginal mucosa is separated from the underlying tissues.
- The peritoneum is cut to get access to the enterocele sac. The enterocele sac's excess peritoneum may or may not be excised.
- To clear the field, the bowel is pushed away from operative field with a large, long mop, and a Deaver retractor (2″) is positioned anteriorly beneath the mop.
- On the side wall another illuminated Sim's speculum is positioned. To get a clear vision of the operating field, when working on the right side, an illuminated speculum is positioned on the left lateral wall, and vice versa.
- Allis forceps can be used to catch the uterosacral ligament, which is visible at the vault on the lateral vaginal wall.
- The uterosacral ligament becomes clearly visible and tactile as you pull the Allis forceps outward by applying traction.
  [If this surgery is performed in conjunction with a vaginal hysterectomy (VH), then traction on the cardinal-uterosacral ligament complex tied up suture will cause the uterosacral ligament to become taut and evident on the lateral vaginal wall.]
- Three suture materials are required: Two nonabsorbable (number "0") and one delayed absorbable (number "0").
- In order to prevent ureteral damage, bites in the intermediate portion of the uterosacral ligament are always taken from lateral to medial.
- Place the initial HULS bite in the uterosacral ligament's uppermost accessible location. Nonabsorbable suture number "0" (polypropylene) is used during the first bite. Medium-sized curved artery forceps are used to grip both ends.
- Same nonabsorbable suture is used for the second HULS suture bite, which is taken between 0.5 and 1 cm below the first one. Medium-sized straight artery forceps are used to grip both ends.
- About 0.5–1 cm below the second HULS bite, the third HULS suture bite is taken using delayed absorbable suture no. "0" (polyglactin). Straight mosquito forceps are used to grip both ends.
- First HULS nonabsorbable suture (polypropylene) punctured the lateral vaginal wall at the vault's right angle on both ends, but it remained inside the vaginal mucosa. Maintain about 5 mm vaginal wall space between the two ends of the suture. Medium-sized curved artery forceps are used to grip both suture ends.

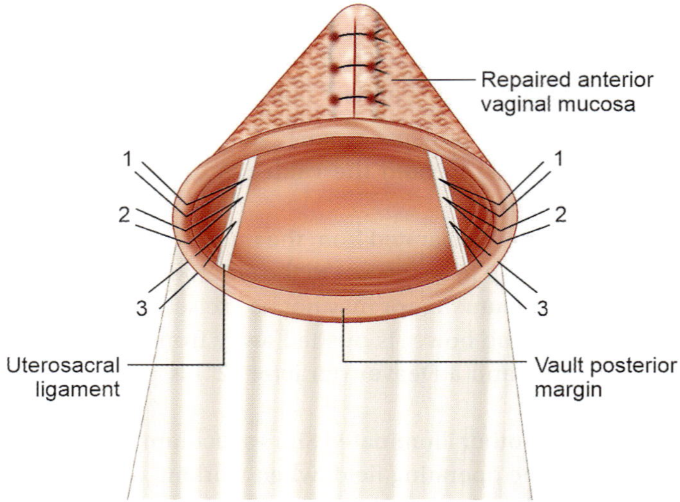

Fig. 1: Intraperitoneal high uterosacral ligament suspension suture: 1 and 2—nonabsorbable, 3—delayed absorbable which only came outside vaginal mucosa.

- Second HULS nonabsorbable suture is secured medially and posteriorly to the first HULS suture in the same manner. Medium-sized straight artery forceps are used to grip both suture ends.
- Third HULS delayed absorbable suture puncture the posterior vaginal mucosa at the vault medial to the second HULS suture and exit the vaginal mucosa. Straight mosquito forceps are used to grip both ends **(Fig. 1)**.
- On the opposite side, the same process is performed.
- Anterior colporrhaphy done.
- Cystoscopy done to rule out ureteric injury.
- Two Allis forceps are used to grip the vault at two angles. The polyglactin no. "0" suture is used to secure one angle.
- Then two ends of the first right HULS suture are then attached to one another. The two ends of the second HULS suture on the right side are then tied. In this way, both nonabsorbable sutures are buried within the vault.
- Continuous interlocking sutures are used to restart vault closure.
- First and second HULS sutures of the other side are tied to their corresponding counterparts as the vault closure suture approaches the other side.
- Vault has been closed. The right side's third HULS suture is now tied up with its ipsilateral counterparts, then left side's third HULS suture is tied up in the same manner.
- The vault is visible in the end, suspended high in the vagina.

EXTRAPERITONEAL HULS

Invented by Professor Peter Dwyer and Fatton B of Australia. This technique was shown for treatment of vault prolapse which is very rewarding. It devoid of chances of ureteric injury.

In case of vault prolapse:

- By looking at the indentation on either of the vault's apex, one can determine where the uterosacral-cardinal ligament (USCL) complex attaches.
- A midline incision is made. Vaginal mucosa is separated from the underlying tissues.
- Dissection is continued laterally into pararectal space to uncover the remains of USCL complex on the side wall of the pelvis, posterolaterally. Exerting strain on the reflecting vaginal mucosa makes it easier to sense these ligaments.
- The bladder and ureters can be kept out of the operating field by using an anterior Breisky-Navratil retractor or a Landon retractor. A delayed absorbable monofilament polydioxanone suture (0 or 00) is placed through the indicated ligament.
- A second stitch made of the same material is placed on the USCL complex above the first suture while the first suture is being pulled.
- On the opposite side, the same thing is repeated **(Fig. 2)**.
- Anterior colporrhaphy and posterior colporrhaphy/colpoperineorrhaphy done, if needed.
- Bilateral suspensory sutures are inserted through the vaginal mucosa and emerge at the newly formed vaginal apex.
- Each of the four suspensory sutures—two on each side—is fastened to its corresponding counterpart **(Fig. 3)**. The new vaginal apex is now positioned high within the vagina.

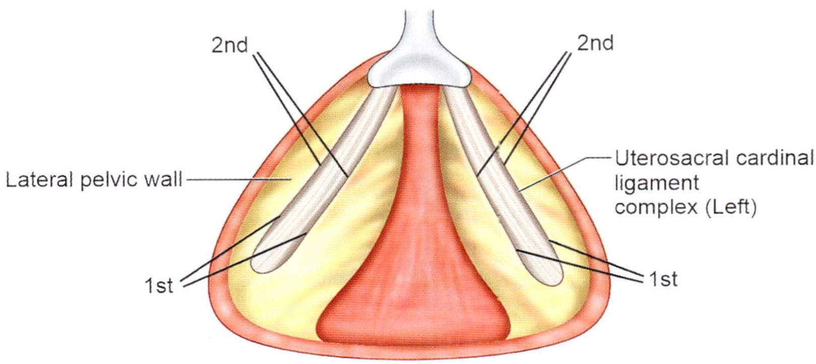

Fig. 2: The uterosacral cardinal ligament complex receives all four suspension sutures.

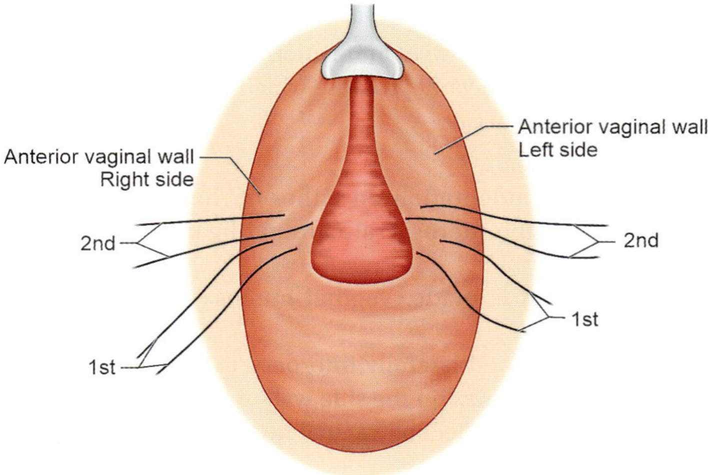

Fig. 3: The suspension sutures (4) are placed outside the vaginal mucosa and identified as the first and second of their respective sides.

PROCEDURE FOR PREVENTION OF VAULT PROLAPSE

- In order to prevent vault prolapse, authors developed new technique of extraperitoneal high uterosacral ligament suspension during vaginal hysterectomy employing the cervix as a traction mechanism (Mani's operation).
- Inverted "V" incision is performed on the anterior vaginal wall and semicircular incision is made on posterior vaginal wall.
- The vaginal mucosa is separated from the underlying tissues. Using Allis forceps, the cervix is gripped and drawn outward to the right.
- A dry gauze is taken on the tip of thumb. On the left side, the thumb is positioned where the anterior and posterior incisions meet. The left cardinal uterosacral ligament complex is exposed by pushing the vaginal mucosa upward laterally.
- We can reach the intermediate section of the uterosacral ligament by simply peeling off the vaginal mucosa from the underlying tissue and exposing it for roughly 5–6 cm **(Figs. 4 and 5)**.
- Pulling the cervix outward toward the left side accomplishes the same thing for the right side.
- Retractors placed for better exposure and pushing bladder and ureters away from the operative field.
- Through right uterosacral ligament's highest exposed portion, a nonabsorbable suture (polypropylene No. 1 or 0) is passed from medial to lateral (first HULS suture). Both the ends are held with straight medium sized artery forceps.

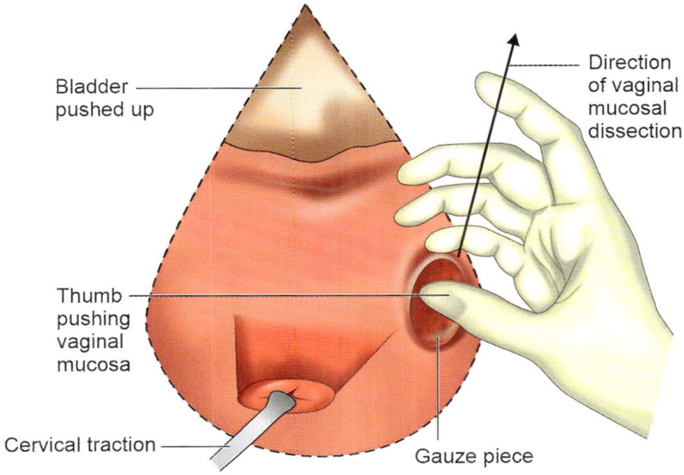

Fig. 4: Exposure of left uterosacral ligament. Cervix is pulled toward right side with Allis forceps. Gauze piece dissection of vaginal mucosa laterally upward starting at the junction of anterior and posterior vaginal mucosal incision.

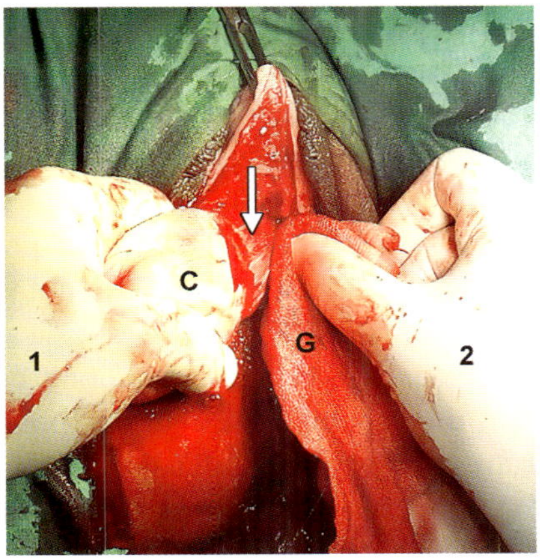

Fig. 5: Exposure of left uterosacral ligament. Traction on cervix toward right side by left hand (1); Gauze piece (G) dissection of vaginal mucosa laterally upward starting at the junction of anterior and posterior vaginal mucosal incision (2); Arrow pointing toward the uterosacral ligament getting exposed.

- Another suture is passed about 0.5–1 cm inferior to first HULS suture in same manner with delayed absorbable suture (polyglactin no. 1 or 0) maintaining cervical traction toward left side (second HULS suture). Both the ends are held with curved medium sized artery forceps.
- Same thing is repeated for left side maintaining cervical traction toward right side **(Fig. 6)**.

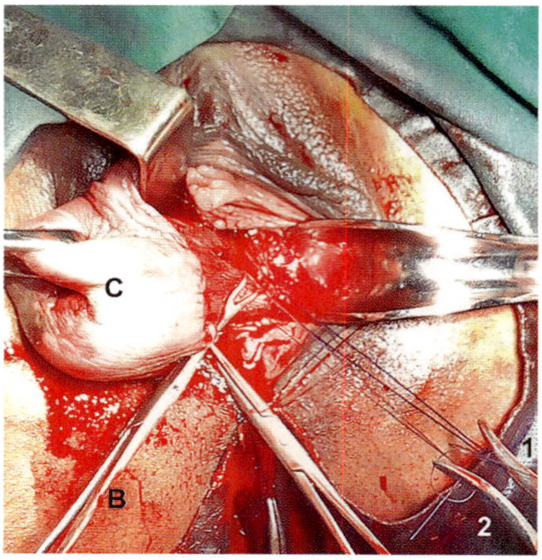

Fig. 6: HULS suture in place in intermediate portion of left uterosacral ligament—(1) First HULS suture (polypropylene); (2) Second HULS suture (polyglactin). Cervical traction toward right side by Allis forceps (C); Exposed left uterosacral ligament is caught hold by Babcock's forceps (B) just for demonstration.

- Next usual first clamp of vaginal hysterectomy done. One suture end is brought outside the vaginal mucosa of the vault. Suture ends are held with mosquito forceps. Vaginal hysterectomy is completed in usual manner.
- Pubocervical fascia is repaired.
- Second HULS suture (polyglactin) lower end pierces the rectovaginal fascia and vaginal mucosa to arrive outside the vaginal mucosa posteriorly medial to the traditional cardinal-uterosacral ligament clamped suture of VH, which was brought outside the vaginal mucosa at the angle of vault.
- Repaired pubocervical fascia is punctured laterally close to the vault area by the upper end of the second HULS suture (polyglactin). Afterward, it penetrates the anterior vaginal mucosa laterally at its neighboring location and exits the mucosa. Medium-sized curved artery forceps are used to hold both ends together.
- First HULS suture (polypropylene) pierces the inner aspect of the vaginal mucosa and the rectovaginal fascia medial to the second HULS suture, but it stays inside the vaginal mucosa.
- Upper end of the first HULS suture (polypropylene) pierces the repaired pubocervical fascia in the region medial to the second HULS suture. This is followed by a bite in the inner aspect of the adjacent vaginal mucosa, which appears superomedial to the second HULS suture. This suture will automatically be placed at the medial aspect of the second HULS suture when it is tied. Avoid piercing vaginal mucosa. Medium-sized straight artery forceps are used to hold both ends together **(Fig. 7)**.
- Same procedure is done on other side.
- Anterior vaginal mucosa is repaired.

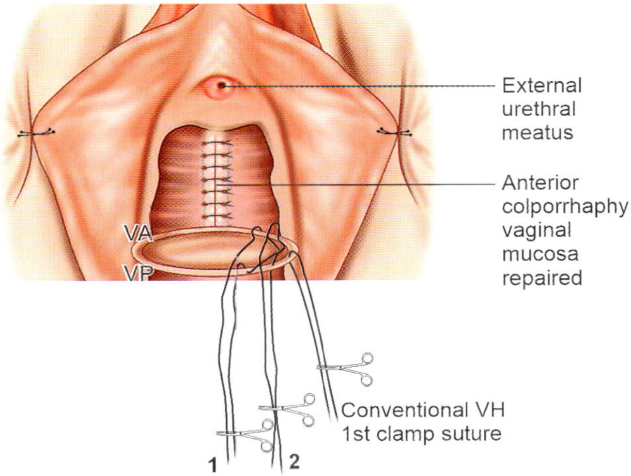

Fig. 7: First HULS (1) suture (polypropylene) are piercing the pubocervical fascia and rectovaginal fascia but not coming outside vaginal mucosa. Second HULS (2) suture (polyglactin) piercing the pubocervical fascia and rectovaginal fascia and coming outside vaginal mucosa. (VA: vault anterior margin; VH: vaginal hysterectomy; VP: vault posterior margin)

- Right angle of vault is secured and suture end is kept long.
- Right first HULS suture is tied with its respective counter parts. Followed by left first HULS suture tying with its respective counterparts.
- Vault closure is completed making burring of both first HULS suture beneath the vaginal mucosa.
- Vault closure suture end is tied with the suture end of conventional VH first clamp of same side which was brought outside vaginal mucosa at the angle.
- Lastly second HULS suture's respective ends are tied together resulting in placing the vault high up in the vagina.

KEY POINTS

High uterosacral ligament suspension is a durable surgical technique to restore apical support in women with vault or uterine prolapse. The uterosacral ligament, extending from the posterior lower uterus to the sacrum, maintains strength with age, making it ideal for suspension procedures. The ligament is divided into cervical, intermediate, and sacral segments; the intermediate portion provides optimal strength while avoiding ureteral injury. HULS can be performed via intraperitoneal or extraperitoneal approaches. Intraperitoneal HULS involves exposure of the ligament through the peritoneum, careful placement of nonabsorbable and delayed-absorbable sutures, and vault suspension while protecting surrounding structures. Extraperitoneal HULS offers a safer route for vault prolapse with minimal ureteric risk. Both approaches aim to elevate and stabilize the vaginal apex, prevent recurrence, and allow concomitant anterior and posterior repairs. Meticulous suture placement, traction techniques, and anatomical awareness are key to achieving long-term anatomical and functional success in prolapse surgery.

SUGGESTED READING

1. Buller JL, Thompson JR, Cundiff GW, Krueger Sullivan L, Schön Ybarra MA, Bent AE. Uterosacral ligament: description of anatomic relationships to optimize surgical safety. Obstet Gynecol. 2001;97:873-9.
2. Dwyer PL, Fatton B. Bilateral extraperitoneal uterosacral suspension: a new approach to correct posthysterectomy vaginal vault prolapse. Int Urogynecol J Pelvic Floor Dysfunct. 2008;19(2):283-92.
3. Fatton B, Dwyer PL, Achtari C, Tan PK. Bilateral extraperitoneal uterosacral vaginal vault suspension: a 2-year follow-up longitudinal case series of 123 patients. Int Urogynecol J. 2009;20:427-34.
4. Pal M, Bandyopadhyay S. Extraperitoneal uterosacral ligament suspension by using the cervix as a traction device. Int Urogynecol J. 2020;31(8):1701.
5. Pal M, Bandyopadhyay S. Modified extraperitoneal uterosacral ligament suspension for prevention of vault prolapse after vaginal hysterectomy. Int Urogynecol J. 2019;30(4):633-7.
6. Pal M. High uterosacral ligament suspension: Extraperitoneal. In: Pal M (Ed). Urogynecology & Pelvic Reconstructive Surgery, 2nd edition. New Delhi: Jaypee Brothers Medical Publishers (P) Ltd.; 2024; pp. 282-7.
7. Pal M. High uterosacral ligament suspension: Intraperitoneal. In: Pal M (Ed). Urogynecology & Pelvic Reconstructive Surgery, 2nd edition. New Delhi: Jaypee Brothers Medical Publishers (P) Ltd.; 2024; pp. 278-81.
8. Vu D, Haylen BT, Tse K, Farnsworth A. Surgical anatomy of the uterosacral ligament. Int Urogynecol J. 2010;21:1123-8.

5 CHAPTER

Sacrospinous Ligament Fixation

Richa Vatsa

INTRODUCTION

Pelvic organ prolapse (POP) is a common condition affecting women, particularly in the postmenopausal period, and significantly impacts quality of life. Apical prolapse, involving descent of the uterus, cervix, or vaginal vault, is a key component of advanced POP. Restoration of apical support is essential for durable surgical outcomes. Sacrospinous ligament fixation (SSLF) is a time-tested vaginal procedure for correction of apical prolapse and is endorsed by major urogynecological guidelines as an effective and safe technique.

DEFINITION

Sacrospinous ligament fixation is a *vaginal apical suspension procedure* in which the vaginal vault, cervix, or uterus is attached to the sacrospinous ligament, usually unilaterally, to restore normal vaginal axis and support. The fixation is most commonly performed to the *right sacrospinous ligament*.

RELEVANT ANATOMY

The sacrospinous ligament is a strong fibrous structure extending from the *ischial spine to the lateral border of the sacrum (S2–S4)*.

Important anatomical relations include:

- Pudendal nerve and vessels (anterolateral)
- Inferior gluteal vessels (posterior)
- Sciatic nerve (posterolateral)
- Rectum (medial, especially on the left side)

Accurate identification of the ischial spine and correct suture placement are critical to avoid neurovascular injury.

INDICATIONS

Sacrospinous ligament fixation is indicated in the following conditions:

- Posthysterectomy vaginal vault prolapse
- Apical prolapse at the time of vaginal hysterectomy
- Uterovaginal prolapse (with or without uterine preservation)

- Recurrent apical prolapse
- Patients unfit for abdominal or laparoscopic surgery

CONTRAINDICATIONS

- Active pelvic infection
- Uncorrected coagulopathy
- Severe pelvic fibrosis or distorted anatomy (relative)
- Inability to tolerate anesthesia

PREOPERATIVE EVALUATION

Preoperative assessment should be comprehensive and guideline-based:

- Detailed history and pelvic examination
- POP-Q staging
- Assessment of all vaginal compartments
- Evaluation for stress urinary incontinence (including occult SUI)
- *Counseling regarding*:
  - Risk of buttock pain
  - Possible recurrence, especially anterior compartment prolapse
  - Dyspareunia
- Informed written consent
- Prophylactic antibiotics as per institutional protocol

SURGICAL TECHNIQUE

Sacrospinous ligament fixation is performed through a *vaginal approach*, most commonly as a unilateral right-sided procedure.

Steps of Procedure

1. Posterior vaginal wall incision
2. Dissection of pararectal space
3. Identification of the ischial spine
4. Identification of sacrospinous ligament medial to the ischial spine
5. Placement of 1–2 delayed absorbable or permanent sutures 2–3 cm medial to the ischial spine
6. Fixation of vaginal vault or cervix to the ligament
7. Closure of vaginal incision
8. Concomitant anterior or posterior compartment repair if required
   Sutures should not be placed too deeply to avoid nerve injury.

POSTOPERATIVE CARE

- Early ambulation
- Adequate analgesia (especially for buttock pain)

- Bladder care and monitoring of post-void residual urine
- Avoid heavy lifting and sexual intercourse for 6 weeks
- Follow-up at 6 weeks and 6 months

COMPLICATIONS

Intraoperative

- Hemorrhage
- Nerve injury
- Rectal injury (rare)

Early Postoperative

- Buttock or posterior thigh pain
- Urinary retention
- Infection

Late

- Recurrent prolapse
- Dyspareunia
- Suture erosion

OUTCOMES

Sacrospinous ligament fixation has demonstrated good long-term outcomes with high patient satisfaction.

- *Anatomical success rate:* 70–90%
- Functional improvement in symptoms
- Lower morbidity compared to abdominal sacrocolpopexy
- Slightly higher anterior compartment recurrence

GUIDELINE RECOMMENDATIONS

According to international guidelines (ACOG, RCOG, and IUGA):

- SSLF is an *effective vaginal apical suspension procedure*
- Suitable for primary and recurrent prolapse
- Unilateral fixation is acceptable and preferred
- Can be safely combined with vaginal hysterectomy and compartment repairs
- Appropriate for elderly and high-risk surgical patients

Various indications and contraindications of SSLF are summarized in **Table 1**.

There are various other surgical techniques for vault prolapse, all compared in **Table 2**.

TABLE 1: Indications and contraindications of sacrospinous ligament fixation.

Indications	*Contraindications*
Vault prolapse	Pelvic infection
Uterovaginal prolapse	Coagulopathy
Recurrent prolapse	Severe fibrosis
High-risk surgical patients	Poor anesthesia tolerance

TABLE 2: Comparison of apical suspension procedures.

Procedure	*Route*	*Mesh*	*Recurrence*
SSLF	Vaginal	No	Moderate
USLS	Vaginal	No	Moderate
Sacrocolpopexy	Abdominal	Yes	Low
Colpocleisis	Vaginal	No	Very low

(SSLF: sacrospinous ligament fixation; USLS: uterosacral ligament suspension)

KEY POINTS

Sacrospinous ligament fixation is a safe, effective, and well-established vaginal procedure for correction of apical pelvic organ prolapse. Proper patient selection, thorough preoperative evaluation, and meticulous surgical technique are essential for optimal outcomes. The procedure offers good anatomical and functional results with relatively low morbidity and is particularly suitable for elderly patients or those unfit for abdominal surgery. Awareness of pelvic anatomy is crucial to minimize complications such as nerve injury and hemorrhage. Addressing all vaginal compartments during surgery reduces recurrence rates. SSLF continues to be recommended as a first-line vaginal apical suspension procedure in contemporary urogynecological practice.

SUGGESTED READING

1. ACOG Practice Bulletin No. 214. Pelvic organ prolapse. Obstet Gynecol. 2019;134:e126-42.
2. Barber MD. Pelvic organ prolapse. BMJ. 2016;354:i3853.
3. Bump RC, Mattiasson A, Bo K, Brubaker LP, DeLancey JO, Klarskov P, et al. The standardization of terminology of female pelvic organ prolapse. Am J Obstet Gynecol. 1996;175:10-7.
4. Carey M, Higgs P, Goh J, Lim J, Leong A, Krause H, et al. Vaginal repair with SSLF. BJOG. 2009;116:138-45.
5. Colombo M, Milani R. Sacrospinous ligament fixation. Obstet Gynecol. 1998;92:803-8.
6. Cruikshank SH, Cox DW. Sacrospinous ligament fixation. Am J Obstet Gynecol. 1990;162:852-62.
7. DeLancey JO. Anatomy and biomechanics of genital prolapse. Clin Obstet Gynecol. 1993;36:897-909.
8. Dietz HP. Pelvic floor ultrasound in prolapse. Ultrasound Obstet Gynecol. 2004;23:80-92.

9. IUGA Committee Opinion. Management of apical prolapse. Int Urogynecol J. 2020;31:3-17.
10. Maher C, Feiner B, Baessler K, Schmid C. Surgical management of pelvic organ prolapse in women. Cochrane Database Syst Rev. 2013;4:CD004014.
11. Morgan DM, Rogers MA, Huebner M. Heterogeneity in outcomes of SSLF. Am J Obstet Gynecol. 2007;197:331.e1-6.
12. Nichols DH, Randall CL. Vaginal Surgery, 4th edition. Philadelphia: Lippincott Williams & Wilkins; 2009.
13. Nygaard I, Brubaker L, Zyczynski HM, Cundiff G, Richter H, Gantz M, et al. Long-term outcomes of prolapse surgery. JAMA. 2013;309:2016-24.
14. Royal College of Obstetricians and Gynaecologists. RCOG Green-top Guideline No. 46. Post-hysterectomy vaginal vault prolapse. Union St, London: Royal College of Obstetricians and Gynaecologists; 2015.

6 CHAPTER

LeFort's Partial Colpocleisis

Sandhya Jain

INTRODUCTION

Pelvic organ prolapse (POP) is highly prevalent among older women, with 11–19% undergoing surgical intervention by the age of 80. However, compared to younger patients, older women undergoing urogynecologic surgery face a 13.6-fold higher risk of morbidity and mortality. Colpocleisis serves as a suitable alternative option for those who are unable to tolerate long extensive surgery and who no longer wish to preserve coital function. The term "colpocleisis" originates from the Greek words *kolpos* (meaning folds or hollow) and *cleisis* (meaning closure). The first documented case of colpocleisis dates back to 1823, when Gerardin described denuding the anterior and posterior vaginal walls at the introitus and suturing them together. However, the technique in use today is a modification of the approach introduced by Leon LeFort in 1877.

SURGICAL STEPS OF LEFORT'S PARTIAL COLPOCLEISIS

Total colpocleisis entails the complete excision of vaginal mucosa, whereas partial colpocleisis (LeFort's modification) preserves the lateral vaginal mucosa on both sides, forming lateral tunnels. In his original description, LeFort proposed creating two trapezoidal sections of the anterior and posterior vaginal epithelium, which were then imbricated to form a tissue platform. The retained lateral vaginal epithelium remains continuous with the cervix, forming two tunnels laterally that facilitate postoperative drainage and provide pathway for any postmenopausal bleeding occurring long after surgery. Surgical steps of this procedure are depicted in **Figures 1 to 6**.

Colpocleisis is a highly effective and low-risk procedure for treating POP in elderly women. Despite advancements in surgical techniques and the growing number of treatment options, colpocleisis remains the least invasive and most durable surgical approach, making it an increasingly favored option. Ideal candidates for this procedure typically have significant medical comorbidities and poor functional

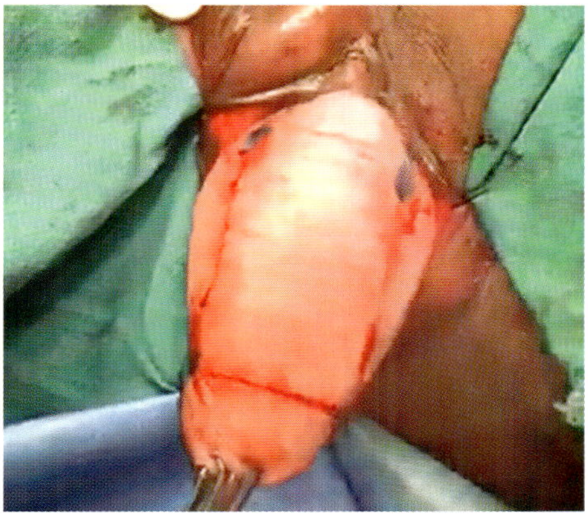

Fig. 1: Rectangular area on anterior vaginal wall is marked.

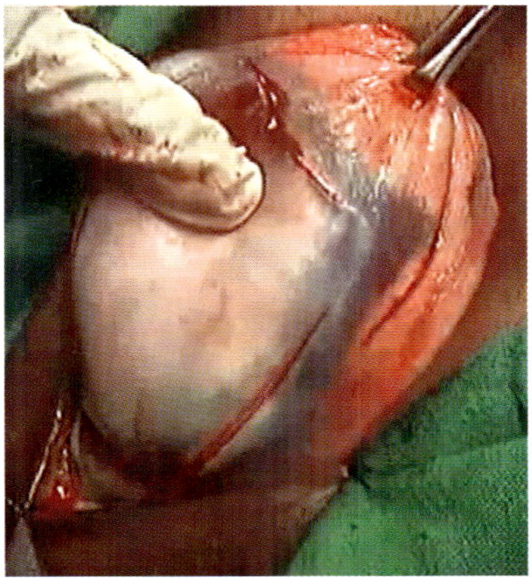

Fig. 2: A mirror image on posterior aspect of cervix delineated with marking pen.

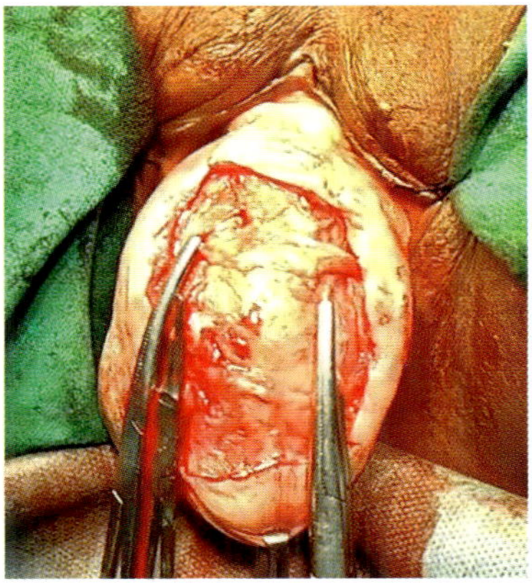

Fig. 3: Anterior flap is removed.

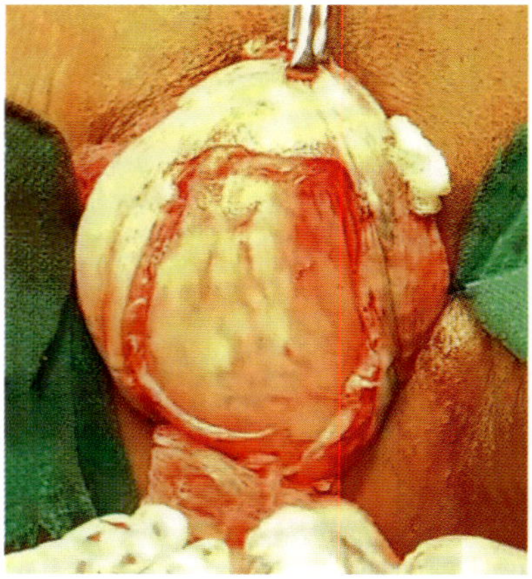

Fig. 4: Posterior flap is removed.

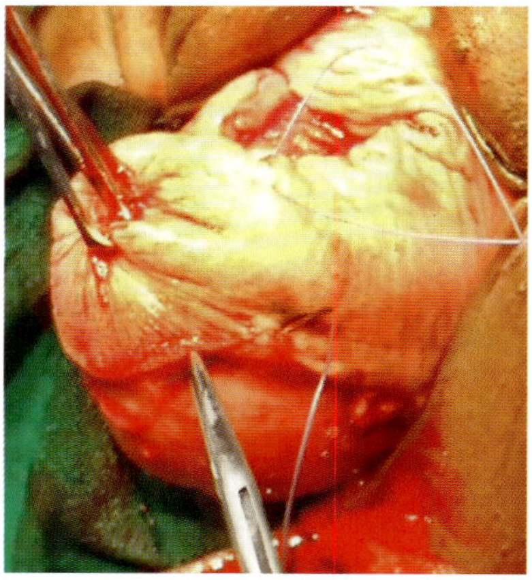

Fig. 5: Anterior and posterior vaginal wall apposition done by serial suturing.

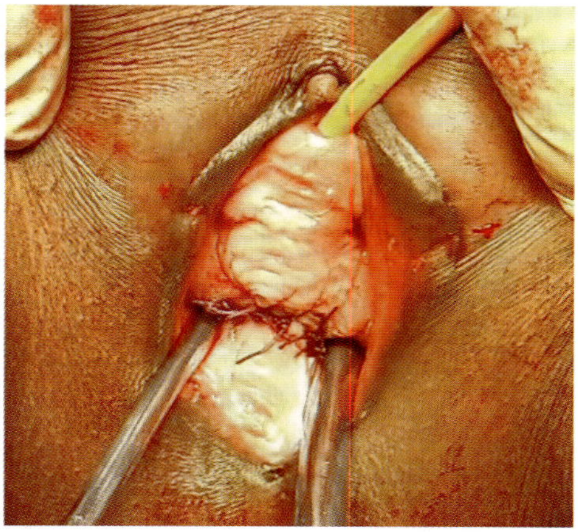

Fig. 6: Two lateral tunnels created as shown by Hegars dilator.

status, making them unsuitable for extensive reconstructive surgery. Since colpocleisis eliminates the possibility of sexual intercourse, it should be considered for patients who do not engage in and do not anticipate any future coital activity. Key benefits of this procedure include shorter operative time, reduced morbidity, minimal blood loss, quick recovery and excellent anatomic success rates. As a definitive surgical solution, colpocleisis significantly improves bowel, bladder and prolapse symptoms, with good patient satisfaction and minimal regret reported. If indicated, sling surgery for stress urinary incontinence (SUI) correction and posterior perineorrhaphy can be performed simultaneously with LeFort's procedure. In one of the largest case series till date, a study by Zebede et al. involving 310 women reported 98.1% anatomic success rate with 92.9% patient satisfaction rate. The complication rate was relatively low at 15.2%, with a mortality rate of 1.3%, indicating that colpocleisis is a safe, effective and acceptable surgical option. The primary drawback of obliterative procedures is the loss of vaginal intercourse. Additionally, the surgery prevents future evaluation of the cervix and uterus for pathological changes, making preoperative assessment for cervical or uterine abnormalities essential. This involves reviewing past Pap smears and cervical biopsies, as well as identifying patients with postmenopausal bleeding who may need an endometrial biopsy or ultrasonography to evaluate endometrial thickness.

Although colpocleisis is a minimally invasive procedure, patients with severe cardiopulmonary conditions that increase anesthetic risk may not be suitable candidates. It is also contraindicated in individuals with cervical or uterine pathology requiring extensive surgical resection and disease staging. The ideal candidate should have a history of negative Pap smears report and no postmenopausal bleeding suggestive of any uterine pathology. Hematoma formation is the leading cause of colpocleisis breakdown or failure, while urinary tract infections are the most common complication. Urinary retention, though uncommon, can also occur.

CONCLUSION

LeFort's colpocleisis is a highly effective surgical treatment option for pelvic organ prolapse in elderly patients, leading to improvements in both pelvic floor symptoms and body image. Its long-term success, high patient satisfaction and low incidence of regret highlight its value as an excellent option for appropriately selected candidates.

KEY POINTS

LeFort's partial colpocleisis is an effective, minimally invasive surgical option for treating pelvic organ prolapse in elderly women who do not desire future coital function. Unlike total colpocleisis, it preserves lateral vaginal mucosa, forming tunnels that allow postoperative drainage and access for any postmenopausal bleeding. The procedure involves excision of trapezoidal sections of anterior and posterior vaginal epithelium, with imbrication and suturing to create a durable tissue platform. It offers benefits such as shorter operative time, minimal blood loss, reduced morbidity, rapid recovery, and high anatomical success. LeFort's procedure can be combined with stress urinary incontinence surgery or posterior perineorrhaphy when needed. Ideal candidates are elderly women with significant comorbidities, poor functional status, and no cervical or uterine pathology. Preoperative evaluation of the cervix and endometrium is essential. Major complications are rare, with hematoma being the leading cause of failure and urinary tract infections the most common postoperative issue. Patient satisfaction is consistently high.

SUGGESTED READING

1. Alshankiti H, Houlihan S, Robert M, Calgary Women's Pelvic Health Research Group. Incidence and contributing factors of perioperative complications in surgical procedures for pelvic organ prolapse. Int Urogynecol J. 2019;30(11):1945-53.
2. Neimark M, Davila GW, Kopka SL. Le Fort colpocleisis: a feasible treatment option for pelvic organ prolapse in the elderly woman. J Pelvic Med Surg. 2003;9:83-9.
3. Pelvic Organ Prolapse: ACOG Practice Bulletin, Number 214. Obstet Gynecol. 2019;134(5):e126-42.
4. Song X, Zhu L, Ding J, Xu T, Lang J. Long-term follow-up after LeFort colpocleisis: patient satisfaction, regret rate, and pelvic symptoms. Menopause. 2016;23(6):621-5.
5. Welch EK, Dengler KL, Wheat JE, Heuer CW, Trikhacheva AS, Gruber DD, et al. Colpocleisis Techniques: An Open-and-shut Case for Advanced Pelvic Organ Prolapse. Urology. 2023;176:252.

7

CHAPTER

Retrieval of Fascia Lata and Rectus Fascia Sling and Autologous Sling Placement for Stress Urinary Incontinence

Richa Vatsa

INTRODUCTION

Stress urinary incontinence (SUI) is defined as the *involuntary leakage of urine during increases in intra-abdominal pressure*, such as coughing, sneezing, laughing, or physical exertion. It results from urethral hypermobility, intrinsic sphincter deficiency (ISD), or a combination of both.

When conservative therapies fail, surgical intervention is indicated. Autologous fascial slings—using *rectus fascia* or *fascia lata*—remain a valuable option, especially where synthetic mesh is contraindicated or undesirable.

INDICATIONS FOR AUTOLOGOUS SLING SURGERY

Clinical Indications

- Intrinsic sphincter deficiency
- Recurrent SUI after failed synthetic sling
- Contraindications to synthetic mesh (infection and erosion risk)
- Patients desiring nonmesh surgery
- Severe urethral mobility
- Neurogenic sphincter dysfunction (selected cases)

Patient Groups Benefiting Most

- Women with previous pelvic radiation
- Patients with autoimmune disorders where synthetic mesh is avoided
- Younger women concerned about long-term mesh complications

TYPES OF AUTOLOGOUS FASCIA

Rectus Fascia

- Harvested through a Pfannenstiel incision
- Dense and strong connective tissue
- Preferred for ease of access during pelvic surgery

Fascia Lata

- Harvested from lateral thigh (iliotibial tract)
- Long, broad, and strong fascial strip

- Useful when rectus fascia unavailable (previous abdominal surgeries)
- Minimal donor site morbidity

RETRIEVAL TECHNIQUES

Rectus Fascia Harvesting

Anatomical Considerations

- Fascia located approximately 2–3 cm above pubic symphysis
- Thickness ~2–3 mm
- Avoid injury to epigastric vessels

Steps in Harvesting Rectus Fascia Sling

1. *Patient preparation:*
    - Supine position
    - Prophylactic antibiotics
    - Foley catheter placed
2. *Incision and exposure:*
    - 6–8 cm Pfannenstiel incision
    - Dissection to anterior rectus sheath
    - Mark a 1.5–2 cm wide and 8–10 cm long fascial strip
3. *Fascial strip retrieval:*
    - Incise sheath carefully
    - Elevate strip using stay sutures
    - Maintain even thickness along the strip
    - Close fascial defect with running absorbable sutures
4. *Sling preparation:*
    - Trim edges
    - Attach permanent sutures (e.g., Prolene) to both ends

Fascia Lata Harvesting

Anatomical Considerations

- Lateral thigh, between greater trochanter and knee
- Thickness variable
- Important to avoid injury to lateral cutaneous nerve of thigh

Procedure Steps

1. *Position and preparation:*
    - Patient in supine position with leg externally rotated
    - Thigh prepared and draped
2. *Incision and exposure:*
    - 3–4 cm longitudinal incision over iliotibial band
    - Sharp dissection to expose fascia lata

TABLE 1: Comparison of rectus fascia versus fascia lata.

Parameter	*Rectus fascia*	*Fascia lata*
Harvest site	Lower abdomen	Lateral thigh
Typical length	8–10 cm	10–12 cm
Donor morbidity	Low	Moderate (pain and hematoma)
Sling strength	Strong	Very strong
Ease of harvest	Easy	Moderate
Ideal for	Concomitant abdominal surgery	Cases with prior abdominal surgery

3. *Graft harvesting:*
   - Mark a 1.5 cm × 10–12 cm strip
   - Elevate with scissors while maintaining uniform thickness
   - Hemostasis achieved meticulously
4. *Donor site closure:*
   - Approximated loosely to avoid tension
   - Skin closed with subcuticular sutures
   - Compression dressing applied

The technique of the rectus fascia and the fascia lata is compared in **Table 1**.

AUTOLOGOUS SLING PLACEMENT TECHNIQUE

Surgical Principles

- Sling acts as a *backboard* under mid-urethra or bladder neck
- Provides support without obstruction
- Works dynamically with increases in intra-abdominal pressure

Steps of Sling Placement

1. *Patient positioning:*
   - Dorsal lithotomy
   - General or regional anesthesia
2. *Vaginal incision:*
   - Vertical midline incision under the urethra
   - Sharp dissection to create bilateral paraurethral tunnels
3. *Passage of sling sutures:*
   - Using a Stamey needle or a similar device
   - Sutures passed from the vaginal incision to the suprapubic incisions
4. *Sling tensioning:*
   - Critical step

   - Sling should be *tension-free*
   - A right-angle clamp or catheter used to maintain appropriate spacing
5. *Fixation:*
   - Sutures tied just above rectus fascia
   - Confirm secure fixation
6. *Closure:*
   - Vaginal incision closed with absorbable sutures
   - Suprapubic sites closed

POSTOPERATIVE CARE

Immediate Care

- Foley catheter for 24–48 hours
- Pain management (NSAIDs/opioids)
- Thigh compression dressing (for fascia lata harvest)

Follow-up

- Voiding trial on postoperative day 1–2
- Avoid heavy lifting for 6 weeks
- No sexual activity for 4–6 weeks
- Assessment of continence at 6 weeks, 3 months, and annually

COMPLICATIONS

Harvest-site Complications

Rectus Fascia

- Seroma
- Hematoma
- Incisional hernia (rare)

Fascia Lata

- Thigh pain
- Numbness over lateral thigh
- Hematoma
- Difficulty ambulating (temporary)

Sling-related Complications

- Urinary retention
- De novo urgency
- Infection
- Vaginal wound complications
- Voiding dysfunction
  Most improve with time or minimal intervention.

OUTCOMES AND SUCCESS RATES

Autologous pubovaginal slings have long-term success rates of 70–90%.

Advantages

- No synthetic material $\rightarrow$ no erosion risk
- Durable long-term outcome
- Effective for severe SUI and ISD

Disadvantages

- Longer operative time
- Higher postoperative pain
- Donor-site morbidity

Still, autologous slings are recommended for women where mesh is contraindicated and in recurrent SUI surgery.

KEY POINTS

- Stress urinary incontinence is involuntary urinary leakage during physical activity due to urethral hypermobility or intrinsic sphincter deficiency.
- Autologous slings remain a vital surgical option, especially for women who are not candidates for synthetic mesh.
- Rectus fascia and fascia lata are the two most commonly used autologous tissues. Rectus fascia is easier to harvest, while fascia lata may be preferred in women with prior abdominal surgery.
- Sling placement involves a tension-free technique where the graft supports the bladder neck/mid-urethra during increases in intra-abdominal pressure.
- Complications may occur at both the donor site and sling placement site but are generally manageable.
- Long-term success rates are high (70–90%), making autologous slings particularly valuable for intrinsic sphincter deficiency and recurrent SUI.
- Patient selection, meticulous harvesting, and appropriate tensioning are the keys to successful outcomes.
- Patient selection, meticulous harvesting, and appropriate tensioning are the keys to successful outcomes.

SUGGESTED READING

1. Abrams P, Cardozo L, Fall M, Griffiths D, Rosier P, Ulmsten U, et al. The standardisation of terminology of lower urinary tract function. Urology. 2003;61(1):37-49.
2. Albo ME, Richter HE, Brubaker L, Norton P, Kraus SR, Zimmern PE, et al. Burch colposuspension versus fascial sling for stress urinary incontinence. N Engl J Med. 2007;356(21):2143-55.
3. Appell RA. Autologous fascial sling for the treatment of intrinsic sphincter deficiency. Curr Opin Obstet Gynecol. 1998;10(5):435-9.
4. Blaivas JG, Olsson CA. Surgical correction of stress urinary incontinence: Pubovaginal sling procedure. J Urol. 1988;160(5):1312-5.

5. Bodner-Adler B, Shrivastava C, Fülöp G. Complications after pubovaginal sling procedures. Int Urogynecol J. 2002;13(4):264-8.
6. Chaikin DC, Blaivas JG, Fitzpatrick CC. Pubovaginal sling surgery for stress urinary incontinence: Long-term results. J Urol. 1998;160(4):1169-72.
7. DeLancey JO, Starr RA. Histology of the urethral sphincter of the female. Am J Obstet Gynecol. 1994;170(6):1713-23.
8. McGuire EJ, Lytton B, Kohorn EI. The value of urodynamic testing in stress urinary incontinence. J Urol. 1993;150(2):322-4.
9. Kobashi KC, Vasavada S, Bloschichak A, Hermanson L, Kaczmarek J, Kim SK, et al. Updates to Surgical Treatment of Female Stress Urinary Incontinence (SUI): AUA/SUFU Guideline (2023). J Urol. 2023;209(6):1091-8.
10. Petrou SP, Brown JA, Blaivas JG. Pubovaginal sling using autologous rectus fascia. Urology. 1999;54(4):642-6.
11. Weber AM, Walters MD. Anatomy of the anterior abdominal wall in relation to rectus fascia harvest. Am J Obstet Gynecol. 1997;176(6):1218-22.
12. Winters JC, Dmochowski RR, Goldman HB. Fascial lata harvest technique and outcomes. J Urol. 1996;155(1):128-31.

8 CHAPTER

Tips and Tricks of Retropubic and Transobturator Routes of Sling Placement

Jai Bhagwan Sharma, Richa Vatsa

INTRODUCTION

Mid-urethral sling (MUS) surgery has become the gold standard for the surgical management of female stress urinary incontinence (SUI). Since the introduction of the tension-free vaginal tape (TVT) by Ulmsten in 1996, several modifications in approach and technique have been developed to improve efficacy and reduce complications. The two most commonly practiced routes for MUS placement are the retropubic and transobturator approaches.

Both techniques aim to provide mid-urethral support without excessive tension, mimicking the physiological support of the pubourethral ligaments. While both approaches have comparable long-term success rates, their complication profiles, learning curves, and patient selection criteria differ. A thorough understanding of pelvic anatomy, surgical steps, and technical nuances is essential for optimizing outcomes.

This chapter focuses on practical tips and tricks for safe and effective sling placement using both retropubic and transobturator routes, emphasizing avoidance of complications and improving surgical outcomes.

STRESS URINARY INCONTINENCE

Stress urinary incontinence is defined as the involuntary leakage of urine on effort, exertion, sneezing, or coughing, resulting from urethral hypermobility and/or intrinsic sphincter deficiency. It affects up to 35–40% of women during their lifetime and significantly impairs quality of life.

Surgical correction is indicated when conservative measures fail. The mid-urethral sling works by providing a hammock-like support to the mid-urethra, allowing dynamic compression during increases in intra-abdominal pressure while maintaining urethral patency at rest.

TYPES OF MID-URETHRAL SLING PROCEDURES

Classification Based on Route of Insertion

- Retropubic approach (TVT)
- Transobturator approach

TABLE 1: Comparison of retropubic and transobturator sling routes.

Parameter	*Retropubic route*	*Transobturator route*
Entry path	Behind pubic bone	Through obturator foramen
Bladder injury	More common	Rare
Groin pain	Rare	More common
Voiding dysfunction	Higher incidence	Lower incidence
Efficacy in ISD	Better	Inferior

(ISD: intrinsic sphincter deficiency)

- Outside-in (Delorme technique)
- Inside-out (TVT-O)

There are differences in retropubic and transobturator routes of sling surgery **(Table 1)**.

RETROPUBIC SLING PLACEMENT: TIPS AND TRICKS

Overview and Definition

The retropubic approach involves passage of the sling from a vaginal incision, behind the pubic symphysis, exiting through suprapubic skin incisions. It provides a more vertical vector of support and is particularly effective in patients with intrinsic sphincter deficiency.

Patient Selection: Tips

Preferable in:

- Intrinsic sphincter deficiency
- Recurrent SUI
- Fixed urethra

Avoid or use caution in:

- Previous pelvic surgery
- Obesity
- Extensive retropubic scarring

Preoperative Preparation: Tricks

- Ensure bladder emptying immediately before trocar passage
- Prophylactic antibiotics
- Proper lithotomy positioning with hip flexion <90°
- Mark suprapubic exit points (2 cm from midline, 1 cm above symphysis)

Surgical Steps with Technical Pearls

Vaginal Incision and Dissection

- Make a 1.5–2 cm midline vaginal incision

TABLE 2: Retropubic sling complications and preventive tips.

Complication	*Prevention strategy*
Bladder perforation	Cystoscopy, proper trocar angle
Hemorrhage	Close pubic bone contact
Voiding dysfunction	Tension-free placement
Bowel injury	Avoid excessive cephalad angulation

TABLE 3: Transobturator sling complications and management.

Complication	*Preventive tip*
Groin pain	Correct trocar trajectory
Mesh erosion	Adequate vaginal closure
Dyspareunia	Avoid excessive tension
Incomplete cure	Proper patient selection

- Dissect sharply until endopelvic fascia is visualized
- Keep dissection close to pubic bone to avoid bladder injury

Trocar Passage: Critical Tips

- Maintain constant contact with posterior surface of pubic bone
- Use non-dominant hand to guide trocar
- Advance slowly with controlled movements

Cystoscopy: Mandatory Trick

- Perform cystoscopy after each needle passage
- Inspect bladder dome and trigone
- Early recognition prevents long-term complications

Sling Tensioning: Tricks to Avoid Obstruction

- Place scissors between sling and urethra (tension-free)
- Ask assistant to remove sheath slowly
- Avoid excessive traction on tape ends

Both the routes of sling placement have its inherent complications, and there are ways to prevent these complications **(Tables 2 and 3)**.

TRANSOBTURATOR SLING PLACEMENT: TIPS AND TRICKS

Overview and Definition

The transobturator approach passes the sling through the obturator foramen, avoiding the retropubic space. It was developed to reduce bladder and bowel injuries associated with retropubic slings.

Patient Selection: Tips

Ideal for:

- Urethral hypermobility
- Primary SUI
- Patients at risk of retropubic complications

Avoid in:

- Severe intrinsic sphincter deficiency
- Prior groin surgery
- Obturator neuropathy

Surgical Anatomy: Trick for Safety

Identify landmarks:

- Adductor longus tendon
- Inferior pubic ramus
- Obturator nerve lies posterior and superior—avoid deep penetration

Outside-in Technique: Practical Tips

- Skin incision at genitocrural fold
- Aim trocar towards ipsilateral shoulder
- Maintain shallow angle to avoid pelvic entry

Inside-out Technique: Tricks

- Start from vaginal incision
- Palpate obturator membrane before puncture
- Keep trocar lateral to avoid bladder injury

Sling Adjustment and Tensioning

- Minimal adjustment required
- Avoid over-tightening to prevent groin pain
- Confirm free urethral mobility

Complications and Preventive Measures

Postoperative Care: Tips

- Early mobilization
- Trial of void after 6–8 hours
- Monitor post-void residual
- Analgesia tailored for groin discomfort in TOT
- Avoid heavy lifting for 6 weeks

KEY POINTS

- Mid-urethral sling surgery remains the cornerstone of surgical management for female stress urinary incontinence.
- Both retropubic and transobturator approaches are effective when used in appropriately selected patients.
- The retropubic route offers superior efficacy in intrinsic sphincter deficiency but carries a higher risk of bladder injury and voiding dysfunction.
- The transobturator route minimizes retropubic complications but may be associated with groin pain and reduced efficacy in ISD.
- Meticulous surgical technique, sound anatomical knowledge, and adherence to tension-free principles are critical for optimal outcomes.
- Mandatory cystoscopy in retropubic procedures, careful trocar angulation, and proper sling tensioning are key technical tricks.
- Individualizing the surgical approach based on patient characteristics ensures maximum efficacy with minimal complications.

SUGGESTED READING

1. Abrams P, Cardozo L, Fall M, Griffiths D, Rosier P, Ulmsten U, et al. The standardisation of terminology of lower urinary tract function. Neurourol Urodyn. 2002;21:167-78.
2. Delorme E. Transobturator urethral suspension: mini-invasive procedure. Prog Urol. 2001;11:1306-13.
3. Karram MM, Segal JL, Vassallo BJ, Kleeman SD. Complications and untoward effects of the tension-free vaginal tape procedure. Obstet Gynecol. 2003;101:929-32.
4. Nilsson CG, Palva K, Rezapour M, Falconer C. Eleven years prospective follow-up of the tension-free vaginal tape procedure. Int Urogynecol J. 2008;19:1043-7.
5. Petros PE, Ulmsten U. An integral theory of female urinary incontinence. Acta Obstet Gynecol Scand. 1990;69:153-60.
6. Richter HE, Albo ME, Zyczynski HM, Kenton K, Norton PA, Sirls LT, et al. Retropubic versus transobturator midurethral slings. N Engl J Med. 2010;362:2066-76.
7. Ulmsten U, Henriksson L, Johnson P, Varhos G. An ambulatory surgical procedure under local anesthesia for treatment of female urinary incontinence. Int Urogynecol J Pelvic Floor Dysfunct. 1996;7:81-6.

9 CHAPTER

Tips and Tricks of Vesicovaginal Fistula Repair

Amita Jain

INTRODUCTION

Vesicovaginal fistula (VVF) is an abnormal communication between the bladder and the vagina. The cause of VVF differs in various parts of the world. The most common cause of iatrogenic VVF is injury to the bladder at the time of gynecologic surgery. Vesicovaginal fistula typically presents with symptoms of continuous urinary leakage from the vagina. This may be as early as 5–7 days after surgery or may be delayed weeks. It is the most common type of urinary tract fistula.

Vaginal repair of VVF should be the preferred primary surgical route because of significantly less blood loss, operative time, decreased use of analgesics, and shorter hospital stays. For a successful vaginal repair, candidates require adequate vaginal epithelium, minimal stenosis, adequate bladder capacity, and no involvement of ureters.

The transvaginal repair is not feasible in many patients due to scarring or narrowing of the vagina, a high location of the fistula, a large (>3 cm) supratrigonal complex fistula or the surgeon's inexperience in transvaginal approach.

The transabdominal approach reduces the morbidity of open approach. It also provides a wider space to work, allows easy access to tissues such as the omentum for interposition, allows repair of complex fistulae requiring ureteric reimplantation **(Fig. 1)** or augmentation cystoplasty, and does not compromise vaginal length.

Minimally invasive approaches like laparoscopic repair has been used for supratrigonal VVF in past. However, this faced challenges like a steep learning curve for laparoscopic suturing and difficulties with access and ergonomics. Although the laparoscopic approach is less expensive, it is technically difficult in a narrow pelvis and with a complex fistula, both with respect to precise dissection of the vagina and bladder and difficult intracorporeal suturing. These issues have been mitigated with the introduction of robotic surgery.

VAGINAL REPAIR

Latzko Technique

The Latzko technique involves a partial colpocleisis without excision of the fistula tract.

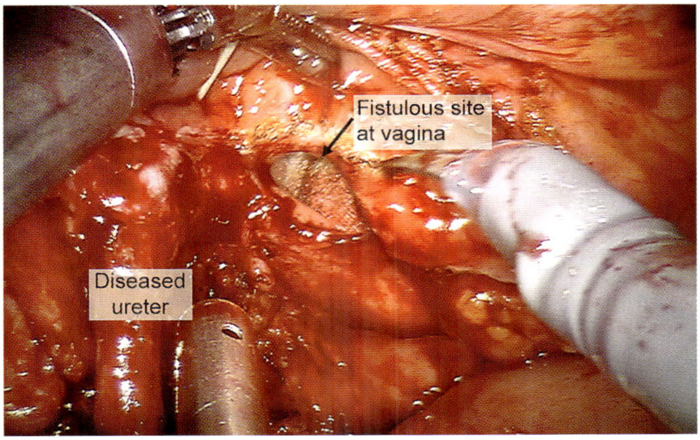

Fig. 1: Fistulous tract with close proximity to left ureter.

Compared with excising the tract, this technique avoids widening of the fistulous tract, bleeding associated with excising the tract, tissue necrosis related to cautery of this bleeding, and injury to the ureter if close to the repair site. In addition, leaving the fibrous tissue lining of the tract may provide support for the repair. Fistulae less than 3 cm can be closed successfully by partial colpocleisis. Reported success of the Latzko repair is between 93 and 100% for primary and repeat repairs without significant problems with vaginal shortening. In a series of 10 patients with VVF repaired by the Latzko technique, none had sexual dysfunction or shortened vaginal length.

Layered Closure

A layered closure is necessary for more distal and complex fistulae. Surrounding tissues are thoroughly mobilized, minimizing tension, and the fistulous tract is excised. Avoid excising excessive amounts of the fistula edges to prevent hemorrhage of the bladder edges and further decreasing the bladder volume. The bladder defect is closed in 1 or 2 layers with 3-0 absorbable interrupted sutures in a transverse fashion near the trigone to prevent kinking of the ureters. The endopelvic fascia and vagina are closed over the bladder using 2-0 absorbable sutures. Alternating horizontal and vertical suture lines prevent the suture layers from lying directly beneath one another. Methylene blue or sterile milk is instilled into the bladder to test the integrity of the repair for watertightness.

Use of various types of suture is described; however, there are no comparative studies recommending 1 suture type over the other. Permanent suture in the bladder may cause calculi and should be avoided. Delayed absorbable sutures such as polyglactin are desirable because of their strength in maintaining a watertight closure.

Martius Flap

Utilization of a tissue flap may be necessary in cases of large, fibrotic, or necrotic fistulae, involving the urethra or when there is inadequate vaginal tissue. The most commonly used vaginal flap is the Martius, a transposition of a labial fat pad with or without the bulbocavernosus muscle. The blood supply comes from the perineal branch of the internal and external pudendal arteries. Success of the Martius flap is 70–100%. Other flaps and reinforcement reported are gluteal fat pads, collagen xenograft, oxidized cellulose, and the cervical lip for juxtacervical VVF closure.

ABDOMINAL REPAIR

Transabdominal-Transvaginal Approach

This approach is specifically useful in complex cases like in patients with a history of prior surgeries whose vesicovaginal space is difficult to dissect or a narrow vagina after radiation treatment. This problem has partly been circumvented by the prone transvaginal approach, but this requires complex prone positioning which is associated with problems in the administration of anesthetics.

Transvesical Approach

The classic transvesical approach described by O'Conor and Sokol involves bivalving the bladder. However, the current trend is towards a limited posterior cystotomy approach.

Minimal cystotomy has the potential to reduce the duration of catheterization and the risk of urine leakage.

Extravesical Approach

This approach for robotic VVF repair was first reported in 2007 by Schimpf et al. In this, repair is done without intentional cystotomy.

TECHNIQUES FOR PREOPERATIVE IDENTIFICATION OF FISTULA TRACT

Sotelo et al. described a technique in which the light from a cystoscope is focused on the fistula while the camera light is switched off in minimally invasive approach. However, the technique involves the need for additional assistance from the patient side cart and side docking to be able to perform cystoscopy.

Others have described tugging a Foley catheter **(Fig. 2)** or a Fogarty catheter placed across the fistula into the bladder. However, passing a Foley catheter is difficult in a small fistula and Fogarty catheter is more expensive. Maintenance of the pneumoperitoneum is done by clamping and tugging

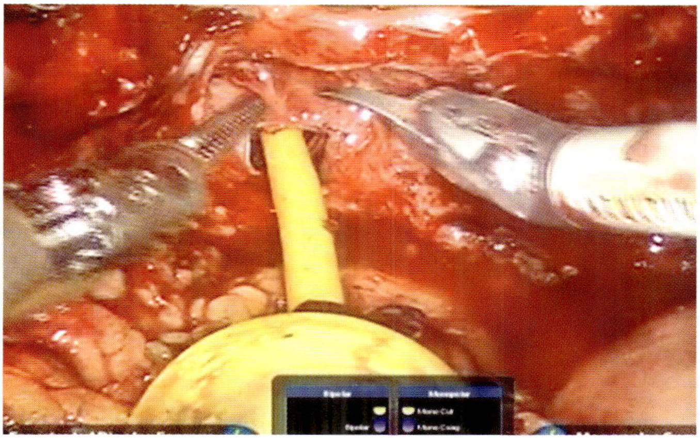

Fig. 2: Identification of VVF tract.

the Foley catheter placed across the fistula to occlude the opening, using an anastomotic sizer modified with an occlusion balloon to manipulate the vaginal apex.

Other option is to place a ureteric catheter across the fistula during cystoscopy and or packing the vagina with a sponge soaked in petroleum jelly. Intermittent tugging of the catheter by the scrub surgeon helps to identify the possible site of the fistula. The ureteric catheter is easy to negotiate over the guidewire and packing the vagina with gauze decreases the leakage of pneumoperitoneum.

TECHNIQUE OF CLOSURE OF BLADDER

Multilayered closure of tissue has been considered important surgical steps for successful VVF repair. Although in various series closure of the bladder in a double layer has been described, a review by Miklos et al. revealed similar success rates for laparoscopic and robotic VVF repair following single-layered or double- layered closure of the bladder. In a study by Sokol et al. in mongrel dogs, double-layered closure of the bladder was shown to be superior to single-layered closure, while another large series describes routine repair of the bladder in a single layer.

INTERPOSITION FLAPS

An interposition flap for VVF works on two theoretical principles: It functions as a barrier and it introduces vascular and theoretically lymphatic vessels that improve tissue growth and maturation. Various interposition flaps have been described in the literature, including omental flaps, sigmoid epiploicae **(Fig. 3)**, peritoneal flaps, and amniotic allograft interposition tissue flaps. The use of biological sealants has also been reported. The use of tissue

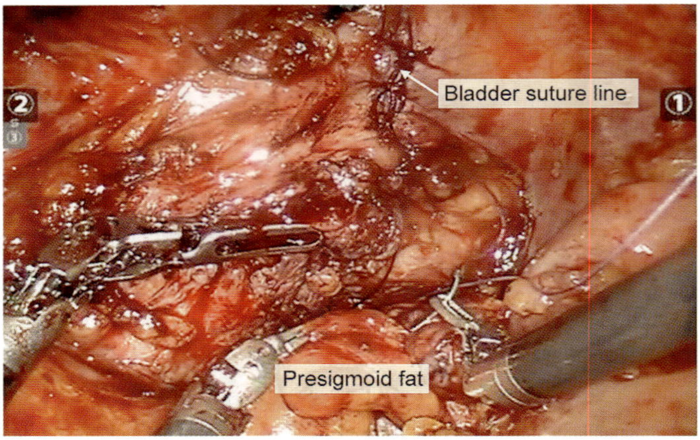

Fig. 3: A vascularized flap of perisigmoid fat for interposition between the two suture lines.

interposition has been questioned in patients who have not undergone radiation treatment. Miklos et al. did not find significantly different cure rates with the use of interposition flaps, and concluded that it is the actual repair of the fistula rather than the use of an interposition flap that determines success, especially in patients with a simple VVF. They shared their experience operating on recurrent VVF with omental flaps reporting a lack of increased vascularity in the previous area of repair and no evidence whatsoever of an interposition graft.

SUCCESS RATE

The success of VVF repair not only depends on the surgical technique but also on the characteristics of the local tissue and systemic conditions that could impair wound healing. The use of the minimally invasive approach for VVF repair has certain well documented advantages in terms of significantly lower operative blood loss, shorter hospital stay, early convalescence and fewer postoperative complications.

Robotic surgery has a similar operating time to the open transabdominal approach. The placement of a suprapubic catheter as practiced in open VVF repair is not deemed necessary in robot-assisted VVF repair because of the excellent hemostasis, satisfactory repair and similar success rates.

CONCLUSION

In developed countries where urogenital fistulas most often result from urinary tract injury during gynecologic surgery, surgeons can prevent fistula formation by using careful dissection and surgical techniques. Especially after hysterectomy, urinary tract integrity should be assessed before leaving the operating room. Success in management is dependent on patient and fistula characteristics as well as surgeon experience.

KEY POINTS

Vesicovaginal fistula is an abnormal communication between the bladder and vagina, most commonly iatrogenic after gynecologic surgery. Patients present with continuous urinary leakage. Vaginal repair is preferred due to reduced blood loss, shorter operative time, and quicker recovery, provided there is adequate vaginal tissue, minimal stenosis, and sufficient bladder capacity. The Latzko technique, a partial colpocleisis without excision of the tract, is effective for fistulae <3 cm, avoiding ureteral injury and tissue necrosis. Layered closure is required for complex or distal fistulae, using absorbable sutures and alternating suture lines to ensure watertight closure. Interposition flaps, such as Martius, omental, or peritoneal flaps, may be used in large, fibrotic, or recurrent fistulae, though success depends more on proper closure than flap use. Transabdominal, transvesical, and minimally invasive (laparoscopic or robotic) approaches are valuable for high, complex, or recurrent fistulae. Success relies on careful tissue handling, patient selection, and surgeon experience.

SUGGESTED READING

1. Bora GS, Singh S, Mavuduru RS, Devana SK, Kumar S, Mete UK, et al. Robot-assisted vesicovaginal fistula repair: a safe and feasible technique. Int Urogynecol J. 2017;28(6):957-62.
2. Dorairajan LN, Khattar N, Kumar S, Pal BC. Latzko repair for vesicovaginal fistula revisited in the era of minimal-access surgery. Int Urol Nephrol. 2008;40:317-20.
3. Dutto L, O'Reilly B. Robotic repair of vesico-vaginal fistula with perisigmoid fat flap interposition: state of the art for a challenging case? Int Urogynecol J. 2013;24(12):2029-30.
4. Genadry RR, Creanga AA, Roenneburg ML, Wheeless CR. Complex obstetric fistulas. Int J Gynaecol Obstet. 2007;99(Suppl 1):S51-6.
5. Kapoor R, Ansari MS, Singh P, Gupta P, Khurana N, Mandhani A, et al. Management of vesicovaginal fistula: an experience of 52 cases with a rationalized algorithm for choosing the transvaginal or transabdominal approach. Indian J Urol. 2007;23:372-6.
6. Kidd LC, Lee M, Lee Z. A multi-institutional experience with robotic vesicovaginal and ureterovaginal fistula repair after iatrogenic injury. J Endourol. 2021;35:1659-64.
7. Ramphal SR. Laparoscopic approach to vesicovaginal fistulae. Best Pract Res Clin Obstet Gynaecol. 2019;54:49-60.
8. Rangnekar NP, Imdad Ali N, Kaul SA, Pathak HR. Role of Martius procedure in the management of urinary-urinary fistulas. J Am Coll Surg. 2000;191:259-63.
9. Sears CL, Schenkman N, Lockrow EG. Use of end-to-end anastomotic sizer with occlusion balloon to prevent loss of pneumoperitoneum in robotic vesicovaginal fistula repair. Urology. 2007;70(3):581-2.

10 CHAPTER

Tackling Complications in Urogynecological Surgery: Prevention, Recognition, and Management

Karishma Thariani

INTRODUCTION

Pelvic organ prolapse (POP) and female urinary incontinence surgery are quality-of-life enhancing surgeries. That framing matters: A complication that might be tolerated after life-saving surgery can be unacceptable here because the patient expects comfort, continence, body confidence, and sexual function. Contemporary urogynecology has therefore shifted from "managing complications" to preventing them through thoughtful procedure choice, meticulous technique, routine intraoperative verification (especially of the urinary tract), and structured postoperative pathways. This chapter focuses on complications in reconstructive POP surgery (native tissue vaginal repairs and abdominal/minimally invasive sacrocolpopexy) and incontinence procedures (synthetic mid-urethral slings and urethral bulking). Complications are organized as intraoperative, early postoperative, and late postoperative events, with practical strategies for prevention, recognition, and management.

PREOPERATIVE STRATEGIES: PREVENTING COMPLICATIONS BEFORE THE FIRST INCISION

- *Risk stratification and optimization:* Address smoking, uncontrolled diabetes, obesity, anemia, constipation, chronic cough, and anticoagulation/antiplatelet therapy. These factors influence infection, wound healing, bleeding, urinary retention, pain, and recurrence. Where synthetic mesh is planned, optimize healing conditions and counsel explicitly that adverse factors can increase the likelihood of exposure or erosion.
- *Vaginal tissue health:* Postmenopausal atrophy increases epithelial fragility and may contribute to wound morbidity and mesh exposure. Where clinically appropriate, optimize vaginal health preoperatively (e.g., topical estrogen in suitable patients) and treat vulvovaginal dermatitis or infection before surgery.
- *Procedure selection matched to goals:* A patient prioritizing minimal invasiveness or rapid recovery may prefer bulking over sling surgery,

accepting lower durability. A patient with advanced apical prolapse and high recurrence risk may accept sacrocolpopexy's distinct risk profile for durable support. Avoid a one-size-fits-all approach; align decisions to symptom burden, anatomy, sexual priorities, and tolerance of re-intervention.

- *Specific consent and complete documentation:* Document baseline voiding symptoms, bowel function, sexual activity, and pelvic pain. Consent explicitly for recurrence, de novo urgency, voiding dysfunction or retention, dyspareunia, and mesh-specific risks where relevant. Clear documentation improves shared decision-making and reduces delayed presentation.

COMPLICATIONS IN PELVIC ORGAN PROLAPSE SURGERY

Intraoperative Complications

- *Hemorrhage:* Bleeding is common in vaginal repairs (paravaginal venous plexus) and may be severe at the sacral promontory during sacrocolpopexy. Prevention relies on dissecting in the correct plane, controlled traction–countertraction, and restrained energy use; excessive thermal spread can trade short-term hemostasis for late tissue necrosis and pain. Management should be stepwise: direct pressure and packing, targeted bipolar energy, clips or sutures, and reassessment of exposure. When bleeding obscures anatomy, repack and re-expose rather than "chasing" a vessel blindly.
- *Urinary tract injury (bladder and ureter):* Bladder injury is associated with anterior dissection and concomitant incontinence surgery. Ureteric obstruction or injury may occur during apical suspension from suture entrapment, kinking, or postoperative edema. Prevention includes identifying landmarks, avoiding deep lateral bites near the uterosacral complex, and anticipating distorted anatomy in redo surgery. Intraoperative cystoscopy is a high-yield safety check; it supports early detection of bladder injury and ureteric compromise. Recognized bladder injuries should be repaired immediately with layered closure and bladder drainage, followed by cystoscopic confirmation. Suspected ureteric compromise warrants immediate assessment and correction (e.g., suture removal/replacement) and urology input for stenting where indicated. The most harmful ureteric injury is the one diagnosed late.
- *Bowel injury:* Although uncommon, bowel injury has high morbidity, particularly during adhesiolysis and promontory dissection. Prevention requires sharp dissection under direct vision, careful entry, and a low threshold for conversion if planes are unsafe. Management depends on immediate recognition, repair (often with colorectal input), antibiotics, and structured postoperative monitoring.

Early Postoperative Complications

- *Voiding dysfunction and urinary retention:* Transient retention can follow prolapse repair due to edema and pain. Persistent retention may indicate overcorrection, hematoma, or obstruction from concomitant anti-incontinence surgery. Prevention includes avoiding excessive anterior tightening, ensuring hemostasis, and using a standard voiding-trial pathway. Management requires early post-void residual measurement, intermittent catheterization protocols, aggressive constipation and pain control, and early reassessment if retention persists beyond the expected window.
- *Postoperative infection:* Includes cuff cellulitis, urinary tract infection, and pelvic abscess. Prevention includes prophylactic antibiotics, gentle tissue handling, meticulous hemostasis (hematoma invites infection), and glycemic control. Management requires prompt review of fever, pelvic pain, foul discharge, or persistent dysuria; culture-guided antibiotics; imaging for suspected abscess; and drainage when indicated.
- *Thromboembolism and ileus:* Older age, reduced mobility, and longer operations increase venous thromboembolism (VTE) risk. Prevention includes formal VTE risk assessment, mechanical and pharmacological prophylaxis tailored to bleeding risk, and early mobilization. Ileus prevention benefits from opioid-sparing analgesia and enhanced recovery principles where feasible.

Late Postoperative Complications

- *Recurrence and failure:* Recurrence is a major driver of dissatisfaction and reoperation. A key technical contributor is inadequate apical support; repairing anterior or posterior walls without restoring the apex invites failure. Prevention includes apical repair when indicated and addressing chronic strain (constipation, cough). Management should be symptom-focused rather than purely anatomical, incorporating pessary, physiotherapy, and reoperation aligned to patient goals and risk tolerance.
- *Dyspareunia and sexual dysfunction:* Dyspareunia may result from scarring, vaginal shortening, over-tightening, pelvic floor spasm, or mesh exposure. Prevention requires tension-free repairs, preservation of vaginal length and caliber, avoidance of excessive excision, and minimal thermal injury. Management includes examination for focal tenderness or exposure, pelvic floor physiotherapy, treatment of atrophy, and multidisciplinary pelvic pain care when neuropathic features or central sensitization are suspected.
- *Mesh complications in sacrocolpopexy*: Mesh exposure or erosion after sacrocolpopexy is uncommon but important. Technique reviews and society statements emphasize prevention: Appropriate lightweight

polypropylene mesh, fixation to well-vascularized vaginal tissue, avoidance of mesh placement over fresh vaginal incisions, and caution with concomitant total hysterectomy, which has been associated with higher exposure risk in expert recommendations. Small, asymptomatic exposures may be managed conservatively with local therapy and observation. Symptomatic, infected, or recurrent exposures often require surgical revision or excision, with the extent (partial versus complete removal) tailored to the location of exposure, symptom burden, and patient priorities. Chronic pain after sacrocolpopexy should prompt evaluation for mesh tension, scarring, nerve involvement, and coexisting pelvic floor myalgia; multidisciplinary management is frequently necessary.

COMPLICATIONS IN FEMALE URINARY INCONTINENCE PROCEDURES

Synthetic Mid-urethral Slings

Retropubic and transobturator mid-urethral sling (MUS) remain widely used for stress urinary incontinence, supported by guideline statements and large evidence bases. Registry-based evidence syntheses report bladder perforation around 0.86–3.6%, voiding lower urinary tract symptoms about 1.47–3.5%, vaginal exposure about 0.2–1.9%, and reoperation up to about 9% in some long-follow-up datasets. Guideline documents similarly describe bladder perforation risk as generally low but variable by technique and setting. These figures support balanced counseling: high likelihood of improvement, alongside defined risks of injury, obstruction, urgency, exposure, and pain.

Intraoperative Complications

Bladder perforation and urethral injury: Prevention relies on correct trocar trajectory, bladder emptying, and controlled passage—especially for retropubic slings. Intraoperative cystoscopy when indicated remains the most reliable method to confirm bladder integrity and permit immediate correction. If perforation is recognized, remove and reposition the trocar and ensure bladder drainage; outcomes are typically excellent when promptly managed.

Early Postoperative Complications

Voiding dysfunction and retention: Many cases improve with time, but persistent obstruction needs timely action. Use structured voiding trials, intermittent catheterization where necessary, evaluate for urinary tract infection and hematoma, and arrange early follow-up. If obstruction persists or symptoms are severe, consider early sling mobilization or incision rather than prolonged catheter dependence; delayed relief risks chronic bladder dysfunction and prolonged patient distress.

De novo urgency: De novo urgency may follow MUS, reflecting altered outlet dynamics or unmasked overactive bladder. Management includes behavioral measures, pelvic floor therapy, bladder training, and pharmacotherapy when needed, with reassessment for obstruction if symptoms are severe or progressive.

Late Complications

Exposure and pain. Vaginal exposure may present with discharge, bleeding, dyspareunia, or partner discomfort. Small exposures may respond to local therapy; symptomatic or larger exposures often require surgical revision or excision. Chronic pelvic or groin pain should be treated as a primary diagnosis: map pain distribution, evaluate neuropathic features and trigger points, begin early multidisciplinary care, and consider revision or removal when pain is clearly mesh-related and refractory, balancing pain relief against recurrent incontinence.

URETHRAL BULKING AGENTS

Bulking offers a lower-risk alternative for selected patients prioritizing minimal invasiveness or those at higher risk from sling surgery. Complications are usually mild (transient retention, urinary tract infection, injection-site pain), but repeat treatments are common and durability may be lower; this should be stated explicitly so that "lower risk" does not become "unrealistic expectation".

SAFETY BUNDLE: PRACTICAL CHECKLIST

Preoperative: Optimize comorbidities, bowel habits, and cough; assess vaginal tissue; document baseline bladder, bowel, and sexual function; counsel specifically.

Intraoperative: Maintain anatomical planes; controlled hemostasis; low threshold for cystoscopy when urinary tract risk exists; minimize thermal spread; verify implants.

Postoperative: Standard voiding trials; early mobilization; constipation prevention; rapid review pathways for fever, persistent retention, severe pain, hematuria, or foul discharge.

CONCLUSION

Complications in prolapse and incontinence surgery are rarely random. They largely revolve around predictable biology (tissue quality and healing), predictable anatomy (urinary tract proximity and presacral vessels), and predictable decision points (procedure choice, tensioning, and intraoperative verification). A prevention-first pathway—paired with rapid recognition and decisive management—reduces morbidity and protects the core aim of pelvic floor surgery. Symptom relief, functional outcomes, and patient priorities should guide management of recurrence rather than anatomical findings alone.

KEY POINTS

- Chronic pelvic pain and dyspareunia after urogynecological surgery require early recognition and multidisciplinary management and should never be dismissed as minor or psychological.
- Mesh-related complications are uncommon but potentially severe; prevention depends on patient selection, tissue optimization, appropriate mesh choice, and precise surgical technique.
- Adequate apical support is critical in prolapse surgery; failure to address the apex is a leading cause of recurrence.
- Postoperative voiding dysfunction should be managed using structured protocols, with early intervention to prevent chronic bladder dysfunction.
- Urinary tract injury remains one of the most preventable serious complications; selective or routine intraoperative cystoscopy should be considered a safety tool rather than an optional step.
- Meticulous respect for anatomical planes and restrained use of energy devices are central to preventing hemorrhage, tissue necrosis, and late pain syndromes.
- Most complications in prolapse and incontinence surgery are predictable and modifiable through careful patient selection, optimization of comorbidities, and appropriate procedure choice.
- Urogynecological surgeries are quality-of-life procedures; even minor complications can have disproportionate physical, sexual, psychological, and medicolegal consequences.

SUGGESTED READING

1. Carlson K, Andrews M, Bascom A, Baverstock R, Campeau L, Dumoulin C, et al. 2024 Canadian Urological Association guideline: Female stress urinary incontinence. Can Urol Assoc J. 2024;18(4):83-102.
2. Deffieux X, Perrouin-Verbe MA, Campagne-Loiseau S, Donon L, Levesque A, Rigaud J, et al. French national guidelines for clinical practice: Diagnosis and management of complications following pelvic organ prolapse surgery using a synthetic non-absorbable mesh. Eur J Obstet Gynecol Reprod Biol. 2024;294:170-9.
3. Duckett J, Bodner-Adler B, Rachaneni S, Latthe P. Management of complications arising from the use of mesh for stress urinary incontinence. International Urogynecology Association Research and Development Committee opinion. Int Urogynecol J. 2019;30(9):1413-7.
4. Farag F, Osman NI, Pang KH, Castro-Diaz D, Chapple CR, Cruz F, et al. Complications of synthetic midurethral slings. Is There a Relevant

Discrepancy Between Observational Data and Clinical Trials? Eur Urol Focus. 2024;10(4):535-50.

5. Matthews CA, Myers EM, Henley BR, Kenton K, Weaver E, Wu JM, et al. Long-term mesh exposure after minimally invasive total hysterectomy and sacrocolpopexy. Int Urogynecol J. 2023;34(1):291-6.
6. Rovner E, Chermansky C, Costantini E, Dmochowski R, Enemchukwu E, Ginsberg DA, et al. Recommendations of the SUFU/AUGS/ICS Female Stress Urinary Incontinence Clinical Guidelines. Neurourol Urodyn. 2024;43:1753-64.
7. Shahid U, Chen Z, Maher C. Sacrocolpopexy: the way I do it. Int Urogynecol J. 2024;35:2107-23.